Unforeseen Journey

JOHN ROCHE

ISBN:

978-1541116832

Reviews of Unforeseen Journey

"*Unforeseen Journey* by John Roche is a raw and honest account of the his personal experience of caring for his mother in his home for ten years -- including the end of life sequences involved. An emotional testimony, it is the definition of love itself, demonstrated in the care provided, but also shows the stresses and strains put upon the caregiver. As uplifting and satisfying as this labor of love can be, there are also life-changing consequences to the caregiver, including exhaustion and burnout.

Roche's goal is to help other caregivers avoid the negative effect of these feelings and to assure that the family member receives excellent care until the very end of life. The downfalls of informal or family caregiving, along with the motivation and strategies to avoid them, are presented based on the Roche's real-life experiences while caring for his aging mother. Critique: Many members of the 'Baby Boomer' generation are now solidly involved in having to take care of their own aging parents, either in their own home or in a sheltered living facility. Exceptionally well written, organized and presented, it is impressively informative, thoughtful and thought-provoking. A 'must-read' for anyone charged with caregiving responsibilities for an aging parent (or any other family member), this book is unreservedly recommended for personal reading lists and community library collections." — Midwest Book Review

"A captivating story of human nature. It will seize you from the first page and never let you go. Powerful and heartrending as you follow the author on his journey. A story grounded in human nature, a must read for anyone."
— HLH

"A book I couldn't put down—brought up so many feelings. I have to read it again more slowly and over a long period of time so I can soak it up —hit the spot for sure." — B. Dunne

"Knowing many who have undertaken this task, some well and some not, this was a book needing to be written. It's obvious *Unforeseen Journey* is a book written by someone who had a profession, children, AND 24-hour care of someone he loved, his mother, leaving precious little time for himself. For those never having had both the joy and the burden of caring for a family member, it's a thought-provoking glimpse of what doing something like this involves, yet possibly not fully able to relate. To those living this experience, it touches every human emotion you may have or may be feeling and will understand it completely. I would recommend this book to all, but particularly to those facing a similar situation now or in the near future. You will get a clearer understanding of the emotions that come with caregiving and then will find valuable resources and information to avoid some of the stresses that come with this formidable task. Thumbs up all the way. I have purchased additional copies to provide to friends in or near this same situation. Makes a great and valuable gift." — Avid Reader

"A well written, insightful, first-person account of the rewards, trials and needs of one being the sole caregiver for a family member. An excellent primer for anyone contemplating this route or a wake-up call for those already committed to this endeavor. Many helpful resources are also included." — Pamela S.

"Have you ever questioned whether you were giving the best caregiving and support you could for your loved one? Have you as a caregiver ever felt helpless or hopeless in the face of stressful repetition and/or suffering almost too unbearable to witness? Have you felt despair in wondering if, at the end of the day, you did well or screwed up? Read Mr. Roche's book. It's going to touch you. It's going to make you feel what you felt when you were tired and cranky and struggling to get through. It's going to make you want to weep when you think of your own particular moment of decision; when, overcome with fatigue and frustration, you failed to think through something ....with damaging results. As I read this book, I thought of my own caregiving experiences and all the ways I contributed to my sister's quality of life in her last years. I acknowledged my own on-going torment of that instance when I, like so many others, felt I let her down; when I felt I let myself down and didn't do the best I could have done. Then I tried to put it in perspective, the same perspective I see as truth for this author. We are human, we make mistakes, but if not for the family caregivers what kind of quality of life would our loved ones experience? In simple reality, what we have done and what Mr. Roche did is the most loving and noble thing a person can do for someone they love. Only when we recognize this truth in the book might we let ourselves off the hook. John Roche has given us a plethora of resources to assist us. Follow his wisdom and his advice....get help and stay healthy. You, and the person you care for, deserve it". — CS

"Well written from the heart and right on as far as what you go thru as a caregiver, excellent" — Avid Reader

"I really enjoyed reading this book! I literally finished in 2 days! Very powerful and emotional! I really learned a lot from reading this especially since I was a caregiver for two young girls with special needs." — Avid Reader

"I have looked for books on the subject but never did I expect to find and read a story of raw emotions! I have read many of the chapters repeatedly, only to relive many of my own feelings. I truly wish I had this book prior to caring for my own family members. It is so very informative and honest. I highly recommend the read for those caring for their own family members or employed caregivers. We will all need care at some point in our lives and preparation is so important in making many difficult decisions. Thank you to the author who shared his personal and valuable story!" — Avid Reader

"This was not a technical, heartless manual about how to take care of a family member but a truly intimate look into the struggles one son had while caring for his elderly mother. Anyone who is considering taking on the daunting task of family caregiving should read this book first."
— Supima

As I sat down to read this book I really didn't know what to expect. In the first 50 pages I was blown away with the raw emotion John had written about. I finished the book in just two days, reading in between work, school, and home chores. I personally have not had this exact experience but this book has taught me a lesson with my own job. Working with kids is no walk in the park, and sometimes I find myself talking in a certain tone or treating my kids in a different manner than I would have in my first year of teaching. The term "burnt out" is a real thing that not many Americans know about or know how to take care of. For the 10 years John was caring for his mom, he went through many hardships not many people knew. I love the way this book is written and I would highly recommend it to anyone who is a caregiver for their loved one, or just wants to read a story about true emotion of caregiving. Job very well done!" — Avid Reader

"What an insightful variation of this author's feelings of being the caregiver to his mother as she ended her journey here on earth. I was my fathers caregiver the majority of the time prior to his death. This book truly helped me realize that I was not alone when it comes to the feeling of guilt associated with the caregiving for a parent during the tail end of their life." — Avid Reader

"This book makes no bones about the positive and painful sides of caretaking, the way the story needs to be told, honestly. The story makes me want to know more, yet is also enough in its cautionary approach. The author should be applauded for this raw truthful story. Thank you for sharing your mother's life and passing with us. It resonates" — Pat

"Brutally honest. Bravely vulnerable. Beautifully powerful. Immensely helpful." — Avid Reader

TABLE OF CONTENTS

A WORD TO FAMILY CAREGIVERS

If you feel that caregiving tasks previously done with ease now require extra motivation and energy to complete, you need to read this book.

If the compassion you once had is waning and you find yourself cutting corners to complete caregiving tasks, you need to read this book.

If you feel that you are approaching the end of your rope and you are overwhelmed due to stress and exhaustion, you need to read this book.

Most importantly, if you are just beginning the work of caring for another human being, you need to read this book. It will not prevent the above-mentioned scenarios from happening, but it will allow you to tolerate them and survive. Challenges are coming your way. Help will be needed. The help starts here.

PREFACE

Caring for another human being certainly requires patience and a good heart. Knowledge and skill are also needed to meet the daily challenges of caregiving. Unfortunately, this very important job often receives little training or preparation.

Assuring the safety and health of a family member, at a time of need, is perhaps the ultimate way of exhibiting love for that individual. Whether this responsibility is a choice or necessity, the demands of caregiving will significantly influence the life of the caregiver. This fact must be acknowledged.

Caring for my mother was a gift for me. It wasn't heroic. It was the right thing to do. I don't deserve a medal. The memories I have of Ma, being present at her death, and sharing the whole experience with family are my rewards and a beautiful tribute to her life.

I made mistakes caring for my mother. Some will say I'm just being hard on myself, but I was there. I know. Complete honesty is expressed here. The details and emotions of this experience may be hard to understand or accept and may even be considered reprehensible by some individuals. I didn't understand many of my own feelings at the time.

My ignorance about caregiving and the effect it would have on me, altered the care I provided for my mom. The person I became was very different from the son who began caring for Ma ten years earlier. I am convinced that this unforeseen and unfortunate transformation could have been prevented.

I am not over the loss of my mom and I shouldn't have to be. Caring for a parent you love and respect so deeply makes it difficult to let them go. Like many things done in life, if we could do them again they'd be done very differently.

My ability for compassionate caregiving was compromised by exhaustion. At the very end, I was not ready to handle something that would change the course of Ma's life. The important lessons I learned should be passed on to others. Otherwise the opportunity to improve the quality of care for someone will be lost. Hopefully, my experience will be a positive influence on the lives of at least one caregiver and their loved one, now or in the future.

Much of what I express is mirrored in the available current literature on informal caregiving. My admiration goes out to those who have taken on the task of caring for a family member. Family caregivers do honorable work, often under trying circumstances, and at a price in terms of their own life.

Informal or family caregivers are family members who care for a parent or loved one in the home. Although the devoted efforts of the informal caregiver can be very rewarding, this noble work can also be detrimental to the quality of life of the caregiver. Definitive steps are needed to avoid this unfortunate outcome. The well-being of the caregiver must be a priority to assure quality, enduring care for the family member.

I'm offering a candid description of my experience as caregiver for my mother. The thoughts and emotions I encountered over this ten-year journey were surprising, given my profound respect and love for her. My mom's care was compromised when I failed to acknowledge the early signs of my own exhaustion and burnout and take the necessary steps to care for myself.

Caring for my mom was a privilege, but I was blindsided by the impact caregiving would have upon me. Knowing ahead of time what I know now would have altered the care my mom received and possibly extended her life. She is my inspiration for this project.

MY ADMISSION

Ma was 76 years old when she could no longer safely live alone. I was 48 when she moved in with me in 2005 and I became her caregiver. It was an honor to care for my mom up until her death in 2015, but it had a tremendous impact on my life.

Prior to beginning this work, I was oblivious to the stresses and strains that were possible when caring for another person. Even if I had been aware, it's very possible I would have been in denial about them affecting me. After all, this was my mother.

My goal was to provide the best care possible for Ma up to the very end of her life. I felt confident and exuberant in my ability to achieve this for her when the journey began in my home. My lack of knowledge about caregiving would come back to haunt me as time passed and I fell short of achieving my goal.

I did not appreciate the effect caregiving was having upon me until my temperament began to change a year or so into Ma's stay with me. I was becoming tense and irritable. I didn't realize how important these signs were or how they would eventually affect the care I provided. The years passed, ten in all, before her death. While family and friends believe Ma received excellent care, this was not the case always.

My mom had physical disability most of her life. She suffered a stroke when she was only thirty-two years old and another when she was fifty-five. Both strokes affected the left side of her body. She could walk up until the age of 76 when injuries, due to falls, necessitated a change in her living situation.

I loved my mom for the unassuming, incredibly strong person she was. I will never fully understand the source of her great determination. She was so admired by those who witnessed her desire to remain independent.

When she could no longer live alone, it was a privilege for me to take Ma into my home. For years, it was anticipated that this would occur. The eagerness to care for her was sky-high, and my motives were altruistic. My mom was loved.

Despite my lofty aspirations, the reality of the day-to-day work would test my patience and temperament as the months and years passed. I felt increasingly pushed to the limits of my capabilities. This didn't happen overnight but in a slow incremental manner. Like sand through an hourglass, the loving kindness of my caregiving ability was draining from me.

The ultimate effect of this was a compromised ability to be as compassionate and caring as I should have been at all times. I'm sure my mom noticed this through the tone of my words and actions. It's disheartening to know that the job of caregiving affected my ability to provide the calm, loving care she so deserved.

This is a cautionary essay for the family caregiver. Giving of oneself in the manner needed to ensure the health and safety of a loved on can potentially lead to feelings of frustration, exhaustion, and burnout. But continue on they do, because for most, they simply have to.

I need to express my experiences and feelings during the past 10 years with complete and utter honesty, so that other caregivers can understand the challenges they face. Some of my feelings may seem cold and callous, but the facts are important to understand the issues encountered.

There was a great deal of warmth and goodness in my care for Ma. She was well cared for but things could have been done better. I believe I contributed to one final incident that led to her death.

I am not a professional caregiver or social worker. I am not a psychologist or scholarly writer. What is said here needs to be said or the opportunity to learn will be lost.

To begin with, a letter to my mom. If only she could read this today.

Dear Ma,

I am so sorry. I knew the end would come but that was not what I wanted for you. I accept responsibility for this by not being ready when you needed me most. I wasn't fit enough to react correctly to what happened. You are not to blame. After all our years together, you deserved more.

I'm sorry for not listening to you more and not being more sensitive to the changes happening to your mind and your body. I was blind. It must have been so scary for you to know that things were changing. Even though we lived together, you were alone through much of this because I wasn't paying enough attention. You could not express easily what you were feeling, and I didn't give you great opportunity to be heard by being there for you as a son. If only I could do this over again.

When stressed and frustrated I went ahead doing what I thought had to be done. I should have stepped back, and taken a moment to realize who you were, my mother, and not just anyone I was looking after. This got lost in the wake of it all. I was naive. All I wanted was for you to be well cared for.

It's very sad to feel you gone because I was with you every day. I may have expressed anger and resentment but just please know that was only because I was ignorant. I loved caring for you. Please know that. I should have done better. I can only say how sorry I am. That's not enough, but it's all I can do. Your memory lives forever. Miss you Ma.

Love,
Your Son

CARING

James is a 64-year-old retired special education teacher. He and his wife have two sons, age 27 and 24, both of whom have severe autism. These boys cannot live independently. They require assistance with activities of daily living such as bathing and dressing, as well as supervision to prevent injury.

Mary is 62 years old and shares the duties of caring for her 94-year-old mother with her sister. Their mom has Alzheimer's disease. Mary is responsible for care Monday thru Wednesday and every other weekend. Mary had to quit her job as a county worker to assist with her mother.

Joyce is 61 years old. Her husband Glen is 65 years old. He is a double below-the-knee amputee due to complications related to diabetes. Glen needs daily help with bathing, dressing and donning his prostheses, which he uses to walk short distances. They have been married for 40 years and live in the home where they raised their children.

Louise takes care of her husband Hector who is 71 years old. He had a stroke 4 years ago. They have 6 children. Louise is the primary caregiver for Hector. Hector communicates through hand and facial gestures since he lost the ability to speak after the stroke. He can walk short distances with a cane but needs assistance with all self-care activity.

Maxine is 42 years old and is the sole caregiver for her 14-year-old daughter Sarah who has cerebral palsy and is wheelchair bound. She goes to a nearby school for a few hours a day. Maxine is a single parent and she does not work outside the home.

These fine souls are known as informal caregivers or family caregivers. They do not come from an agency and they receive little if any reimbursement for their work. Informal caregivers allow those needing care to remain in the home and close to family, while avoiding expensive institutional forms of care.

Jane, who suffered a stroke at age 38, due to uncontrolled hypertension, is now 61 years old. At age 53, she had a brain injury from a fall. The stroke and brain injury both affected the function of her left side. She lives in an apartment with her two sons, ages 27 and 29.

Jane needs assistance with bathing and certain aspects of her self-care. One son helps, but reluctantly so. This puts her in an uncomfortable position. She is worried about her need for additional help now and in the future. She is unable to afford professional care, and does not want to depend on her sons for assistance.

Jane "gets it," as she says, that being tied to the care of their mother may be too much to expect of her sons at their age. They have lives of their own and she knows that they will be significantly affected by her reliance on them for the help she needs. She puts her own safety at risk in sparing her sons the responsibility of caring for her.

Caregiving imposes many consequences upon a caregiver. There is the immediate effect that begins from day one when the hands get dirty for the first time and the lower back awakens to the new-found demands. Routines are established and adjustments in schedules are made for meal preparation, feeding and bathing. The caregiver's managing of personal finances and maintenance of the household may be sandwiched between their caregiving duties. There are trips to the grocery store, pharmacy, and doctors. Heavy responsibility can come with the beginning of each new day.

Feelings of reward and satisfaction with what's being provided to the family member or loved one may be strong and motivating as these challenges are met with success. The caregiver proceeds along the learning curve of physically and mentally handling all that needs to be done and, at the end of each day, there is a feeling of 'mission accomplished.'

The latent effects of caregiving are the most ominous. The real impact of caregiving is felt when the road has been traveled for more than just a few miles. Issues of stress and burden can begin to overshadow the initial motives and desires to care for the loved one. Compassion may be replaced by the desire to be finished with what needs to be done as quickly as possible, sacrificing the kindness and softness that once existed.

The caregiver needs to keep this progression in mind as an eventual, distinct possibility. Surprising as it may be, this is a sign that needs a response—an action plan—or it will only worsen.

Help is needed, but it won't appear magically. It needs to be sought after by the caregiver because few, if any, know all that you are going through. This is an important dilemma, and part of the strategy of being a healthy family caregiver.

The effect of caregiving upon the caregiver's life becomes palpable when the caregiver's own health and personal responsibilities begin to suffer. Only those who have given of themselves in this way can fully understand the true meaning of it.

CARING FOR MY MOM

My mom was a very simple person. She had great strength, bundled in sweet softness and modesty. I loved her for her ability to endure for years and years after her stroke without anger or even a complaint. It was a gift to care for her. However, I do not have much sense of accomplishment or feeling of a "job well done."

My motivation to do what was right for her was ingrained in me from the time I was a child, as I witnessed her incredible determination. I had immense desire to help my mom, to eliminate her struggle and provide for her a safe environment without risk for more injury. She had earned that. Bringing Ma into my home was a pleasure and a relief long anticipated.

My career as a Physical Therapist afforded me the knowledge and capability to handle Ma properly. It was my job to deal with people with physical disability, so, naturally, I was the one who should care for her. Ma was wheelchair bound and needed significant assistance and the right technique to move from one seating surface to another. I knew what to do to accommodate her physical limitations.

I feel that it was my fate to take care of my mom. It was the right decision for me to take on this responsibility. All possible options considered, this was the logical living situation for Ma now that she could no longer live alone.

Ma received good care with the help of family and friends. She was included in all family gatherings, and it was great having her involved in the daily happenings at home. Ma's health and well-being were the focus of attention. We had fun together. She could see and experience things she would have never experienced if she hadn't lived with me. Ma's grandchildren were close by and their presence in each other's lives was a joy for all.

It was rewarding to see Ma safe and smiling every day. She had someone to say good morning and goodnight to her. It felt good to eliminate her struggle and make her laugh. Contributing to her health and wellbeing was uplifting. This was the upside to caregiving.

The downside was more subtle and sinister. Caregiving had a delayed effect on my ability to always be patient while caring for Ma. As the years passed, my focus changed from doing everything I could for Ma to getting the essentials done and going on with my own life.

Caring was something I wanted to do for Ma because I loved her. But the work of caregiving over the years fostered unwanted emotions within me. The negative feelings were not toward Ma, but rather toward the work required to care for her and the time it took away from me. This was unexpected and made the work harder.

I didn't feel unappreciated in the work with my mom. I felt irritated with the fact that no one knew the difficulty of it, and how it kept me from living. This is what amplified my frustration with the caregiving process. No one could understand because they weren't there every day to see it and feel it.

I didn't want to complain about it because I wasn't going to change the arrangement anyway, so why stir the water? I carried this inside of me when I should have expressed it. In the end, it influenced the softness with which I handled the most demanding of my caregiving duties.

Stress levels peaked when I felt pulled in too many directions by the regular demands of life in addition to my obligations for Ma. Instead of acting upon these feelings to remedy them, I suppressed them and forged ahead, thinking that was what I needed to do. That was a mistake.

The years passed and I was approaching a breaking point. It's a terrible feeling to be up against something and have no way out. You must proceed even when you feel you can't go another step. Such was the case for me toward the end of my mom's life. I thought that nothing about the situation was going to change and I didn't want it to, so I simply needed to live it out.

The care of my mother was compromised in ways that were in no way abusive but, instead, callous to whom I was caring for. My care of Ma became very unlike what a son should have provided. Soft, sensitive care was lost at times and replaced by a mechanical form of attention I never knew existed in me.

I admittedly lost my patience on occasion, particularly when something happened to delay or interfere with the routine of caring for Ma. Inconveniences or delays meant my life was altered more than it already had been. My tolerance for this wore thin and I became easily annoyed.

The chemistry between two people in a confined space created its own natural form of friction and tension. Differing opinions, tastes, and moods, with the added effect of bad timing, naturally created conflict on occasion between Ma and me. Ma and I would squabble about some of the silliest things, for no other reason than to have something to talk about. However, a larger issue was taking center stage. The demands of caregiving, and the sacrifices needed to meet them, drained my ability to be tolerant and compassionate.

My perspective about who I was caring for, and how I was doing it, was losing its focus. She was my mother; I was her son. The distinction between being a caregiver and a son turned gray. Once I would go the extra mile in assuring little things were done for Ma, because she was my mother. This was replaced by an attitude of taking the shortest distance between two points.

It was this change in the normal mother–son relationship that was most tragic and which dulled my sensitivity. Casual indifference replaced the idealistic desire of doing something good for my mom, all because I failed to act upon the signs that were in front of me.

I needed a break and I didn't take it.

I wasn't completely unaware of my eroding patience and heightened irritability. I could feel it; I felt like a pot simmering on the stove. There were periods of rising anger and frustration, related to caregiving, exacerbated by normal life situations that would bubble up to the surface and pop. Then I'd feel better for a while.

A good laugh, a nice breeze, two hours away at the movies or a simple memory of Ma would defuse the situation momentarily. Then, with another diaper change or Ma's obsession overseeing something that wasn't there, my stress level would rise and cause me to become something other than the type of person I wanted to be for her.

The months and years passed. Cyclical feelings of satisfaction and discontent chipped away at my tolerance for caregiving. There were many times when I wanted to be finished with it.

I shudder now to think of how the resentment and frustration I felt toward caregiving may have seeped its way out through my mouth and hands and into the care of my mother. There, in the moment, there was no alarm from my conscience. I was too hell-bent on finishing what had to be done.

My communication was short at times and my hands lost much of the tenderness they'd had before. This was buffered by fleeting, occasional glimpses of the former relationship between Ma and me: that warm and caring one, where we would laugh or exchange a smile. These flashbacks would ground me and restore my compassion, at least for a short while. The pendulum swung back and forth. Soft and caring one night, short and mechanical the next.

Then I was caught off guard one night, ill-prepared to react properly to something that happened in the bathroom, as I was getting Ma ready for bed, something we had done thousands of times before. This called for my utmost patience and it wasn't there. I was unable to make a quick decision that could have made a difference. Instead, my mom passed away nine days later.

Those who knew of this incident considered it simply an accident. However, if my mind had been in a better place, I possibly could have prevented it from happening. Accidents occur for a reason in most instances. Going too fast, carelessness, poor planning or distraction all can lead to accidents. I feel this "accident" was caused by my ignorance. I was spent, and did not appreciate the impact of this upon my own self. By this time, I was ill fit to be the caregiver I needed to be. I hadn't paid enough attention to what was happening within me. This is the reason this "accident" occurred.

I had the strength and physical ability to care for my mom. I lacked patience for what I was doing. As the years passed, this got worse.

The task of caring for my mom was harder than I thought it would be. I was not smart enough, nor humble enough, to see that I needed help. At the very end, I was out of gas and unprepared to deal with a critical situation that required quick action.

My mom is not to blame for anything in terms of my deteriorating level of patience and compassion. Never taking a break to recharge my batteries and maintain my caring capability is to blame. This was a mistake.

Compassionate caring ability requires the right temperament. You can't bake bread without flour. Proper temperament for the caregiver needs to be nourished, and I believe respite care is the only way to achieve this.

Giving of oneself day after day in the care of another human being without respite care for the caregiver will lead to unfortunate repercussions down the line. Outside family members must be aware of this. It is critical for the well-being of not only the caregiver, but for the health of the one being cared for

My mom's need for attentive care was beyond well deserved. She never took for granted to care or help she received. In fact, she was embarrassed that people were assisting her, humbled that she was served. She would much rather have been left alone to struggle if she had her way, but she was loved way too much for that.

How could it happen that my softness hardened in caring for my own mother as the years passed? How? Why?

The answer is this: I didn't take enough time away to recharge and take care of myself which eventually affected the care I provided. I didn't heed the limits of my own capacity to be a compassionate caregiver. Period. I'm not being hard on myself. This is simply what happened. There is a limit to how far a person can go, and how much they can do without help. I exceeded this to a fault. I didn't know any better.

I'm writing this so that caregivers may avoid what may be a natural path leading to burnout. Caregiving must be punctuated by breaks—timeouts—for the restoration of the caregiver's ability. This is important for all parties related to the care receiver to know.

THE TRUTH AND MY DETOUR

Ma may well have thought it was going to be a temporary situation when she came to live with me. My family and I knew differently. She was wheelchair-bound with left-sided limbs that didn't work. Ma had survived many hits and was now going to be cared for in a way that should have begun long before.

My mom was a sharp, intuitive person, trapped inside a body that could not function well. She was an avid reader and did crossword puzzles every day. Her spelling and word comprehension abilities were amazing. Ma loved talking about Hollywood of the 1930's and 1940's. Her favorite books were biographies, mainly of people from that era and, eventually, I would have great difficulty finding one she hadn't already read.

Conversations with Ma were easy. She had an innocent, unassuming way about her that people loved. You could talk to her about anything very comfortably and she never judged. Shy by nature, Ma always put others ahead of herself. She expressed interest and greatly enjoyed the simple one-on-one conversations at the kitchen table over coffee.

Ma's strokes had affected the left side of her body. Her left arm was nonfunctional, contracted up with a bent elbow and wrist and no finger movement. Her left leg tended to be straight at the knee and a contracted heel cord made the left foot point downward. She leaned to the left always and could never sit up straight. She looked at the world somewhat sideways for many years.

Despite her physical distortion, she had a straightforward practical way of seeing things that made you take notice of her observations and thinking ability. You could never underestimate Ma, even as bashful as she was. That would be when she'd surprise you and she did this often.

Ma came to live with me when she could not manage to live alone any longer. I attended to Ma's basic needs and she had social stimulation unavailable while living alone. After several years of expecting this to happen, it was now a reality. She was with me and I was happy about it.

My attention to Ma may have been a bit overboard to begin with, but it settled down as our first year together proceeded. Routines were established and we got used to the fact that we were once again living under the same roof after some 30 years.

We were on a positive path. My goals and idealistic views of what this was going to be like were coming to fruition. Having Ma close put a certain spring in my step that I didn't have before. I felt I was doing something right. There was work involved but it was satisfying. Ma was being well cared for.

The flame of my enthusiasm began to flicker after a year or so. Varying emotions began to exist as I came to realize the impact of caregiving for someone within my personal space. The lack of freedom and privacy that came with this new living arrangement began to hit home. My disposition began to vacillate between happy and grumpy as I proceeded through my daily duties.

I was a divorced dad with three young children ages 15, 13 and 11. I wanted to spend as much time as possible with them. Having Ma close at hand was a blessing, yet it added to the load I was trying to manage. Reflecting back on this now I feel my plate was overloaded. There was a lot to do and not enough time in a day to do it.

I sensed something was happening inside of me. Almost as if a faint alarm was going off deep down, but I never took a moment to analyze the cause. There were no timeouts available, no time for reflection. I was heading down a path that was not in the best interest of either Ma or myself.

Another surprising trend was taking shape. The line between caregiver and son was losing its definition as time passed. The distinction between these roles faded. This was a most unfortunate happening. I was with Ma as her caregiver more than I was as her son. The imbalance pushed the closeness we once had to the back burner. The work it took to clean, dress, and nourish Ma damaged my ability to be close to her. I blame the caregiving process for the barrier that developed between us, but I accept responsibility for not doing anything about it.

If I had been able to make the distinction between the two roles, it would have helped improve the situation. Caregiving distorted our relationship. Was I a son or simply someone caring for my mom? It felt like the latter more and more as years passed. Something got lost along the way. Losing the perspective of this relationship was sad and had many implications over time.

Four or five years into Ma's stay with me I began wondering what Ma's life expectancy would be. How long could a person survive in her situation? She was past 80 now and hadn't walked for 5 years. Wouldn't pneumonia or the flu strike at some point, simply for natural reasons? Deep down, what I was wondering was how long I could go on being saddled with this responsibility.

Alzheimer's disease appeared when Ma was about 80 years old. She was aware of a mental decline in herself before anyone else was. Recall of words, memories, and people's names became challenging for her. The swings between fluency and confusion were subtle, inconsistent and confusing. I would wonder, could it be a bladder infection, dehydration or simply a bad day? I saw a gradual slide but did not fully appreciate the onset of Alzheimer's disease, about which I knew very little. In fact, at one point Ma had to tell me, "You know I'm getting Alzheimer's."

25

The early signs of Alzheimer's disease went undetected by me for several reasons. First, I didn't know what these signs were. There were memory issues or slight bouts of confusion on Ma's part that I simply blew off, thinking she was in her eighties and that's what I should expect. Difficulty in recalling the names of her grandchildren was, in hindsight, one of the first pieces of memory to fade. She was embarrassed by this and, I'm sure, this caused her concern about her thought processes.

Secondly, I was too busy to be sensitive to subtle changes in Ma. There was a lot to be done between Ma, the care of the house and errands, etc. Some days were better than others. I was more patient with Ma when outside influences were minimal or I didn't have to mow the lawn. On those days, I was a better caregiver. Most the time though, particularly on the weekends, there was a hectic pace to get things done and I couldn't slow down enough to be in step with Ma.

The third reason I didn't detect the early changes of Alzheimer's, was that I didn't want to. I feared Ma's mortality. I feared watching her decline. I didn't want to make it official by admitting that she had Alzheimer's disease.

Ma's daily routine changed due to increasing bouts of confusion and physical weakness. Ma was once able to propel her wheelchair around the house very well. Then she needed to be pushed, so she wouldn't get lost or stuck. She loved to watch old-time movies before her attention span deteriorated and she began sleeping for increasing periods of time during the day. Interaction with the hired caregiver diminished. The conversations with Ma were what I and the caregiver missed the most. The softness, the practicality of her way was charming. It was sad to see this decline.

These changes weren't consistent. There were good days and bad. The ups and downs were hard to follow. We theorized about whether Ma was getting enough sleep, or whether she was possibly dehydrated. Just when we thought maybe we had something figured out, there would be an aberrant reaction and we would be lost again.

She had been a meticulous and careful eater all along. A tremor in her right hand began to interfere with food going directly from the plate into her mouth. Control of her saliva and food became poor. Feeding herself became slow and very messy. I could sense Ma's frustration, but she handled hers so much better than I did my own. It became hard to watch her feed herself. I would often take over and feed her, just to assure that she would get food in a reasonable amount of time.

Surely, she was struggling with what was happening. I wish I would have shown more softness and understanding toward her. It wasn't that she didn't want to eat or answer a question. It was because she couldn't make the connection between a thought and an action as fast as I wanted her to. But I was often hell-bent on finishing my work with Ma so I could go on to do my things. "Come on Ma, here we go." "Ma, are you ready?" "Let's go Ma, we don't have all day." I was usually 2 or 3 steps ahead of her, out of sync.

These changes associated with Alzheimer's disease didn't happen from one day to the next, but rather over a 5-year period. Ma was very sharp her first 5 years with me. You could tap into her sense of humor easily and make her smile. She actively participated with her own care and was very observant about her surroundings. Then, very slowly, short-term memory began to fade, followed by gradual step-downs in other abilities.

It was when things took longer for Ma to do that the challenges of caregiving began to ramp up. I became impatient with the delays associated with what was happening in Ma's head. Her reaction time to a question or command increasingly slowed. Waiting for her to open her mouth for food when I was ready to give it became a chore. When I would give her an option or choice between two things, I would often make the choice for her because I didn't want to wait.

This didn't happen all the time, but on just enough occasions to know I was becoming low on fuel for caregiving work.

When my patience varied so drastically from one day to the next, I would wonder why to myself, but it never became a call for action. I never changed anything in terms of getting help. One day I would be kind and jovial with her. The next I would be cranky and irritable. There were many contributing factors to this including work and relationship-related stress and the amount of rest I'd had. I now believe the primary factor was that I never built a consistent break into the routine of caregiving.

My respite from caregiving responsibility came when I went to work. I was gone most of the day while the hired caregiver took care of the day's activities. When I got home, the baton was passed to me but I was tired and not at my best. I still had a job to do. By the time the weekends were over and I had two full days of caregiving behind me, I was more than ready and willing to return to work on Monday.

My interaction with Ma was often minimal in the evenings after work. I'd walk in and say "Hi Ma," and she'd respond "Hi John." I'd ask her if she needed anything and she invariably said no. Ma's mental decline in the later years allowed me to be in the same room with Ma but not have to communicate. I had been talking and listening to people all day at work and I relished quiet when I got home. So, there we would be, sitting eight feet apart, in silence except for the television.

In the later years, Ma was frequently asleep when I got home. She would respond to the touch of my hand on her knee by opening her eyes briefly. Then she would return to sleep.

Sometimes she would be staring blankly as I approached her. She would mouth the words, "Hi John." The caregiver would give me an update as to how Ma ate that day, and any other unusual activity.

Ma resting comfortably when I got home was a luxury for me because I could do other things, or simply nothing at all. I wish now that I would have had the ability to sit directly next to Ma at this time when I got home just to spend a few quality minutes with her, or just hold her hand. No need to entertain or talk but just to be there with her. This is a regret I have. Instead she was often left alone.

Ma's deteriorating strength, vision, and memory affected what little independent wheelchair mobility she had left during the last two years. She began to get stuck in corners or end up down a hallway and not be able to figure her way out. She would get lodged against a piece of furniture or stuck between the stove and the island in the kitchen. When I returned home from being out somewhere and found her in a corner, I would ask her how long she'd been there. She always said, "a minute or two." I knew differently.

I began leaving Ma in her recliner chair for longer and longer periods of time because I knew she was safe there. It was padded, deep and impossible for her to get out of on her own. This would give me a break. Her immobility prevented her from getting up and into trouble. I used this to my advantage while running errands, doing things outside and around the house or visiting others. The recliner became something that allowed me some opportunity to live life, at least a little.

Occasionally, I would watch her try, over and over, to get out of that chair, but I wouldn't do anything about it. I knew she would fail, so I just let her continue. Eventually, I figured she would give up, but her persistence was incredible. It was hard to watch this so, inevitably, I'd attempt to adjust her, pull her up, or use pillows for support. But she would soon return to her attempts to wiggle out of that chair. I would ask if she wanted to get up into her wheelchair and she would respond that she wanted to see what was in the box across the room. Of course, there was no box. So, I left her in the chair.

The last five years of Ma's life were a transition from a sharp, interactive person to someone frequently lost in the fog of Alzheimer's disease. I didn't feel the sadness or sympathy I should have felt watching this because there was always the work of caregiving to be done. However innocently this occurred, caregiving, in essence, spoiled my ability to be with Ma as her son, and for us to enjoy the soft moments we once had.

On Sunday night, November 8, 2015, an event occurred in the bathroom as I was getting Ma ready for bed. This was a critical point for Ma in her final decline toward death. Our routine in the bathroom, that had developed through the previous 3,650 or so nights of preparing Ma for bed, went wrong. I feel this could have been averted if I had been a healthier caregiver.

Preparing Ma for bed every night was a very important part of our relationship. This process would start at around nine o'clock at night. The day was over and the TV was finally off. There was quiet. For the first time in the day, we would be able to sit within inches of each other without distraction.

It was hard to muster up the energy to do what was needed for Ma at the very end of the day. Some nights were harder than others to answer the bell at nine o'clock, but it had to be done. This bathroom time was the best time to talk to Ma and enjoy a few moments of the illusive mother-son relationship. A brief sense of compassion would even return to my hands and voice.

Every night I would roll Ma into the bathroom in her wheelchair and place her on the toilet. Then I would leave to put her dirty diaper in the trash and get a new one along with her pajamas. I'd give Ma a few minutes alone in the bathroom for privacy before returning to care for her.

It was during this brief interlude, between leaving Ma alone and returning to care for her, that my mind would go off on tangents. I would think about things that I never anticipated thinking of when I started caring for Ma ten years prior. How much longer can I go on like this? How much longer can Ma go on like this? When will I get my life back? Why can't anyone else know what this is like?

The amount of time I took before returning to Ma in that bathroom depended on my stress level. Sometimes I would purposely try to find other things to do just so I wouldn't have to go back in there. It was the mere thought of the physical work of cleaning and changing Ma that would repel me from getting back in there promptly.

The hardest part was just getting to the bathroom door. It was as if the doorknob was hot. Figuratively, I really had to push that door open at times, to get to my job. Then the sight of Ma sitting there, waiting patiently for me, would soften me at least temporarily.

My attitude should have never progressed to this point. There was so much good about having Ma with me, but it was tarnished by the work that had to be done every day. She never once complained about the time I left her there on the toilet.

I'd sit on the edge of the bathtub next to Ma's side while I attended to her. There I could look into Ma's eyes and feel for where she was. She had gotten the most out her body and she was tired after fighting off the effects of those strokes for 50 years. Ma was such a beautiful, strong woman to me, making it all the harder to watch her decline physically and mentally.

It was during these 15 minutes or so in the bathroom that I'd feel the most compassion for Ma and the most frustration against the caregiving process. I'd look at Ma and think how much I'd miss her when she was gone, but still look forward to the day when this work would be done. The contrast in feelings was confusing and caused guilt within me. There was a polarity to my thinking, like two animals fighting with each other in my head over not wanting to lose Ma, yet wanting this job to be over.

The fact that it was the end of the day and my tolerances were diminished was certainly a factor. Depending on the happenings of the day and my fatigue level, I would either be my normal self or someone else. When not myself, I'd be less communicative, more in a hurry, and forgetful of the fact that this was my mom. If things didn't go well when I sat down to clean and change Ma, I would revert to something cold and mechanical just to be done with the job as quickly as possible. This was the dichotomy. I wanted to be with Ma. I just didn't want the work.

To remedy my tension over the work that had to be done, we would often go through our routine in the bathroom in silence. This was my way of dealing with the trials of handling the wet diaper and dressing Ma around her uncooperative limbs. I would put my mind somewhere else just to get through the physical aspect of caring for Ma, a defense mechanism to keep myself from completely losing it.

I loved Ma and loved being with her, but it was the chore of her care that wore me down. Like a runner with worn out shoes or a carpenter with a dull saw, my draining bucket of compassion was affecting the work that had to be done. Where was the relief?

I hated her stroke and the stiff limbs that made my work harder. I knew this epitomized my selfishness, in that Ma was the one who had to live with it all those years. But it was difficult to separate my frustration from her hardship. It took much self-persuasion to see that her 50-year plight with the aftereffects of stroke was far more difficult to bear than my intermittent frustration with her limbs. Even so, I failed more often than I succeeded.

When silence didn't reign, and my tolerance permitted, I would bring up a news item from the day or something that was going on with the kids. She would take interest and maybe make a comment, maybe not, but I knew she was listening. This would make me feel there was still a connection. When she responded verbally, it was particularly gratifying.

Those brief moments of coherence were so enjoyable, like the old days. She made occasional, funny little comments, about my slow achy movements or my coughing noises, that would make me laugh. She always assumed I was sick, and I'd have to convince her I wasn't. She was showing concern.

I greatly enjoyed that time in the bathroom with Ma when we communicated, but I never told her so directly. I never told her I was lucky to care for her. There were so many missed opportunities as the weeks, months and years passed to say what I wish I could have said.

I should have told her, at least once while in that bathroom, that taking care of her was not a burden, that it was what I wanted to do so she could be safe. I never told her that and I never told her I loved her during that nighttime routine. Something was in the way, and it was the work I was doing.

The moments of clarity and alertness became less frequent as time passed. I didn't take advantage of the alert times nearly as much as I should have. My chances were there but I didn't take them. The grind of caregiving had interfered with my ability to talk with Ma as a son should have.

Ma would sometimes make comments as if I were trying to hurt her. It was insulting at first and would make me mad briefly. Then I'd reason that this was part of her decline. Still, this would push me one click further toward the finish line of wanting to be done with it all. This progression of thought didn't happen overnight. It was slow, glacial-like at times, but nonetheless real.

I don't remember ever feeling depressed so much as I felt just plain irritated. I could never do what I wanted to when I wanted to do it. There would always have to be a plan made, or precautions taken to leave the house. I felt drained by the repetition of it all without having a break. Where was the person with the whistle to call a timeout?

If I ever felt down or melancholy, it was after family left, after visits for birthdays or holidays. It was a bit rewarding for me to have people see that Ma was alive and well. But after the party was over, it was back to the same old routine.

The bitterness I felt at times wasn't toward Ma. It was due to Ma's clothes not going on or coming off as easily as I wanted them to, or the wheelchair not rolling properly. In a larger and more significant way, it was because the rest of the world didn't know or appreciate how hard it was to sacrifice my needs and desires to care for someone who would, at times, criticize me for how I was doing it. This was the source of the anger. If someone had told me on occasion that they knew this was very difficult, it would have made a big difference.

Looking back, the effect of caregiving on my behavior was most prominent at the one-year mark and again around the seven-year mark, with many peaks and valleys in between. The one-year mark was significant for all the adjustments made, when I was first realizing the impact of this on my life. The freedom and privacy previously enjoyed were gone. I needed to be home at a certain time and there was work to be done when I got there. Life was different.

Over the next five or six years, I got used to things and settled into what I was doing. We plugged away and managed to do what needed to be done. There were a lot of distractions. Ma was taken on outings to parks, restaurants, and the kids' sporting events. Ma's faculties were still intact and she could participate well in a family get together.

My caring tolerances sputtered around the seven-year mark as I was becoming increasingly exhausted with the job of caregiving. The spikes in my discontent were becoming more intense and more frequent. Ma was going through the changes related to Alzheimer's disease, and her physical ability was declining. The "sacrifices" I was making were weighing me down. I wished, with increased frequency, that my job was done. Yet, I had to help Ma more because she was unable to do many things she once did by herself. Feelings of increased burden settled upon me.

I hope she didn't see, hear or feel my unhappiness. My words of frustration and the mechanical way I handled her may have indicated that she was a burden. I should never have said things out of frustration, but I did. She deserved better.

I rarely just sat with her for a moment and held her hand. I never found the right words to tell her it was a pleasure to care for her. Even if I didn't say anything to her, I should have at least sat next to her, instead of eight feet behind and to the left, all those nights in front of the television.

In those later years, just when I felt like I'd hit my absolute limit, something would happen to calm the water. Opening that bathroom door and seeing her there waiting would restore my softness, at least temporarily. The soft feel of her palm or our eyes meeting would awaken my tender demeanor, and I would remember that this was my mom. The duration of my positive attitude would be determined by what got in my way next when caring for Ma. Occasionally, the slightest snag in our routine would set me off, wanting to be done all the faster.

Conflicting thoughts would occur as to whether what I was doing for Ma was the right thing versus putting her in a facility. On one hand, I enjoyed her and felt the years she spent with me were worthwhile. On the other hand, my aggravation got the best of me at times as I morphed into something other than the caregiver I originally intended to be.

I felt pressure to appease the wishes and needs of others for my time, despite feeling they knew nothing about what it took to care for another human being in this way. I certainly wanted to participate in life like others did, but I couldn't. Offers to go here or there and do this or that had to be turned down because I could not take the time away from home.

The totality of the situation, at the seven-year mark, sank in: I was burned out with the routine, tired of being pulled in different directions, and tired of watching Ma struggle with boredom and decreasing function. It was a rising crescendo of stress in my last three years with her. I regret not fending this off. I didn't have a strategy and it was too late.

In the last six months, Ma became very sensitive to quick movements or sudden changes in position. She was afraid and showed signs of anxiety. I didn't have the time or the inkling to explain to Ma every move required for her care. Thus, she would often act as if she thought I was trying to hurt her.

She would say, "Why do you do that?" or "Why are you like that?" She would grab my arm and quickly release it as if in disgust or anger. I was trying to be gentle and get her ready for bed as best I could. This would take a little more out of me if I was not in a caring frame of mind. When I was sympathetic it was much easier to let this comment go. Those times became harder to come by.

I was not as comforting and reassuring with Ma about her decreasing faculties and increasing anxiety as I should have been. Her capacity to see, hear, feel, and process was still there, just delayed or intermittent. It was hard to tell at the time what got in and what didn't. She was not to blame. As I would learn later, much more of what I said or expressed landed in Ma's conscious mind than what I thought.

I would say in trying to ease her fears, "No problem Ma. We got this covered." But this was on a good day for me. I didn't say this often enough. As the years passed, my desire to get things done was tripped up by the delays in Ma's processing capability. Less and less was I able to slow down and be in sync with Ma.

There were many nice, satisfying days with Ma when she was around family and friends. The interaction was fun. Then, after everyone was gone, the demands of the caregiving role would ruin my disposition and I would become irritable again. I wanted to just be done with the work, out of that bathroom, and into my own space.

I can't get the time and opportunity back now to say what I should have said to Ma as her son. I should have gotten help. I feel I was unprepared, undisciplined for the process. I feel I should have had a coach or someone I could have been accountable to for what I was doing. Where was the manual on how to do this, how to cope?

I very often let what was happening on my cell phone interfere with what I had to do with Ma. A ball game on television (and not necessarily a good one), or some mindless application on my phone kept me from having to think about what was next in terms of caregiving. Anything to distract myself became an easy path to follow. I'd get up and help Ma with something to drink, but there was little interaction. Back to my phone or the remote I went.

Caregiving affected all aspects of life. My work, my responsibilities to my kids, as well as the general maintenance needed for life were all affected by my role with Ma. I would put things off, like bill paying and house maintenance, simply because I didn't have the motivation to do anything else after doing what I had to do for Ma. I was told at times that I was spread too thin. That turned out to be an understatement.

Also affected was my relationship with my significant other, Darlene, who is an integral part of this story. We met about a year into my care of Ma and became boyfriend-girlfriend. Our relationship had its ups and downs during Ma's stay with me. It was not easy for Darlene to be involved with me in my caregiving role. I had a lot to do and Darlene had to wait, on many occasions, until I finished these things. She was of tremendous help to me but I never showed appreciation for the time constraints placed on her and the patience she displayed. Our relationship was both benefited and hurt by having Ma in my home.

My health trended downward during those 10 years. I was 20 to 25 pounds overweight, eating to relieve stress. I took medication for diabetes and hypertension. My activity level was poor. There was no desire to exercise after feeding or changing Ma. There were simply too many other things to do. No time was afforded for personal maintenance and this was damaging to me as an individual.

After all that has been said, I still do not regret the decision to move Ma in with me. That was my calling. She was not able to live alone and we didn't want her in a nursing home. All I wanted was for her to be well cared for.

Somewhere along the way, I veered off the desired path. I'm not perfect, but ignoring my limitations and not paying attention to the signs that I needed a break were serious mistakes. Eventually, this affected the care I provided for Ma. I had no guide and went blindly into this work, as so many others have done.

The story of Ma and I is important to relate. Those who find themselves in a similar situation should know in advance what impact this may have on their life. Lasting, compassionate care of their loved one depends on it.

ONE MOTHER'S LIFE

My mom and dad met at a picnic somewhere in Oakland, California, on a Sunday afternoon, in the summer of 1956. Jack was 28 and Charlotte was 27. They were married within a year and eventually settled into a home on the San Francisco Peninsula in 1958. This is where family life would begin for Jack and Charlotte.

I was the first born in 1958, followed by my sister in 1960, and my brother in 1961. Needless to say, my mom was very busy her first few years of marriage. My dad was a pharmacist and owned his own pharmacy at the time. He was a hard worker and spent seven days a week at his store.

My dad also had a disease: Alcoholism.

His love for the drink affected Ma's life from the very beginning of their relationship. Three children in the first four years of marriage would be enough, but he was a workaholic/alcoholic. There wasn't much time for him to help Ma at home.

Ma began to have headaches in 1962, within a year or so of giving birth to my brother. She was 32 years old. According to medical records, she experienced numbness, on the left side of her body, that would come and go. Then one day, the numbness didn't go away. She had suffered a stroke. The exact cause of the stroke was never determined. Weakness in her left hand and leg resulted. It was a cruel twist of fate for such a beautiful, young woman who was so busy with three young children.

It's possible she may have simply broken under the strain. My dad was gone much of the time, either at work or hanging out in bars. I was only four years old when she had this stroke. My sister was three and my brother one. Something had to give.

My dad worked long hours and came home drunk regularly. Business at my dad's drug store was slowly going downhill. I remember conversations between my parents about giving the store up. He spent much of his time in the bars attempting to drown his worries. There was one located across the street from his drug store. Easy access meant extended periods of time away from home.

Time marched on and the stroke didn't keep Ma from raising the three of us kids as we grew into our school years. Ma worried at night about when dad would get home and what shape he'd be in when he got there. She would watch the clock--seven, eight, nine o'clock. If he didn't show, she would call his favorite watering holes and ask that he be sent home. How humiliating this must have been. "It's time to come home," she would plead into the phone with desperation.

I remember sitting out on the curb in the dark with Ma one night when I was about 10 years old. We were waiting for a cab to take us to the store because Dad had not gotten home in time. Ma was sobbing and talking about things I did not fully understand. I only knew she was sad and angry and I didn't like seeing her in that way.

It wasn't until I was in junior high school that the heartache and stress Ma was experiencing became clearer to me. Financial hardship kept Ma on edge. She worried about money a great deal. There was constant conflict between mom and dad over the drinking. She wanted it to stop and begged my dad to change things.

Dad would have fits of rage if things weren't right when he got home. She shielded us from the drunken meanness by telling us to go outside or to our rooms. When sober my dad was a helpful, sensible person. When drunk, he was nasty and abusive. Ma protected us from him in those situations.

We never saw any outward affection between our parents. I cannot remember my mom and dad hugging, kissing, or holding hands.

There was a bond between them though. When the alcohol didn't interfere, they seemed to mesh together. As I recall, there were quiet interactions, smiles, and the normal, humorous aggravations between two married people. I remember my dad scratching his head in perplexity, with a grin on his face over something Ma would do.

There had to be something good present for Ma to hang in there the way she did. In the 1970's divorce was a much more difficult option than it is today. As far as we know, Ma never considered it. What would she do and where would we go? She had a physical handicap and three young children.

Mom and dad had both been only children. Now, together they had three kids to manage and perhaps this created their need to lean on each other. Whatever it was, there was definitely something about them to make one think they were a good couple.

As far as parenting, my mom shouldered most of the load since dad wasn't around a great deal. Ma made us do chores and our homework. She took us to parks and lakes. When we needed a ball cap, she was the one to get it for us. Ma even taught us how to play the piano.

My brother related the story of how Ma would put away one dollar here and there with the goal of going on a little trip somewhere. I remember these trips very well. It was always the four of us: Ma and us kids. Dad was working. There were trips to the Russian River and to Lake Tahoe. Just three to four days of time together. Nothing like Disneyland, camping or boating trips. They were simple, little vacations with just the four of us in a small cabin or hotel room for two or three days.

We would usually buy our food at the store on these trips and prepare it ourselves rather than eating out. Money was always tight. Not being home must have been good for Ma in some way. She planned long in advance for these little trips. They were important and I remember them fondly.

My mom's parents were a big part of our lives when we were young. My brother and sister and I would spend a week or so at their home during the summer. I'm sure Ma appreciated the break. I never knew if Ma and Dad took trips or went out to dinner together while we were away. What I do remember is my dad gone most of the time, but the three of us having a normal childhood because of Ma's efforts and the help of our grandparents.

When my dad's business closed, he looked for jobs in and around the San Francisco Bay area. We eventually moved 45 miles across the bay, during the summer between my sophomore and junior years of high school. I think Ma may have looked at this as a fresh start. Maybe the drinking that had been so harmful to our family would be less in a new environment away from the previous hangouts and drinking buddies.

That was not the case. My dad, lacking the control he had enjoyed when he was self-employed, became frustrated with his new job. He had disagreements with management, continued to drink, come home late at night and do the foolish things alcoholics do. Eventually he lost that job.

My mom was devastated. I remember her wondering aloud if he would ever find work again. He found part-time jobs from then on, but never eight to five, Monday through Friday work with a regular paycheck. I'm sure he was demoralized by this and worried about providing for his family. Although he would have denied it, he had an illness with a strong grip on him. My mom's parents helped us financially and this must have been a further insult to Dad's pride.

This was a very stressful period for Ma. She had three kids in their early teenage years, which is not an easy phase of life under normal circumstances. My grandparents, who must have been conscious of the strain my mom was under, moved to be closer to us. Their support was a big help to my mom and our family.

Meanwhile, Ma's uncooperative body, as the result of her stroke, affected her function. Her left hand was impaired to the extent that she could not grasp or release objects well. It was easy to see that her left leg lagged behind the right when she walked. She was much slower than everyone else and it was obvious that all her movements required extra effort.

The stroke must have affected her self-image as a woman but we never knew it. The only makeup she wore was lipstick. Her only jewelry was a gold band wedding ring. I don't remember her ever buying anything for herself. She made many of her own clothes, working with patterns, pinning material and using the sewing machine, all with impaired use of her left hand. There was never anything she couldn't do. She plodded along just a bit slower than the rest.

Dad continued to drink and stay out late. I would worry about what would happen when he got home because he was often verbally abusive to my mom when he was drunk. I'd go out to the kitchen, if there was conflict, but Ma would just turn and quietly tell me to go to bed. Dad would crack open another beer, and demand that Ma make him something to eat. Or he would sit in his chair in a drunken stupor for the next few hours.

I would later hear him bump his way down the hallway in the middle of the night on his way to bed. In the morning before school, we would find him reading the newspaper at the kitchen table, smoking a cigarette, and drinking a beer for breakfast.

My dad tried to find work but had little success. He probably didn't leave the most flattering impression with his last full-time employer, so a good reference was hard to get. He did some part-time work here and there which seemed to give him a bit of a lift.

One night my dad came home very late and, as he parked, I could hear the tires screech loudly against the curb. The engine turned off and the door opened. As soon as the door closed I heard him hit the street with a thud. I didn't want him to be seen lying out there so I rushed past Ma who was standing at the door. I pulled him up the sidewalk and into the entryway of the house. He was a big man and my anger fueled my strength.

He was out of it, asleep, drunk. I remember Ma staring down at him. She was clenching her right hand and saying, "Damn it to hell." Ma's frustration made me even angrier. She turned away and went into the kitchen. I followed her there but I didn't know what to say to her. She told me to just go to bed. I remember this moment as if it were yesterday. He would lie there all night. We had to step over him to get out the door to leave for school the next day.

When I got home from school that afternoon I learned my dad had been taken to the hospital with a broken hip. The hip must have broken when he fell out in the street. Another scar of drunkenness. This required surgery to repair and some rehabilitation afterward. He came home walking with crutches.

Of course, Ma took care of my dad when he got home. He needed help dressing, getting food, etc. and she did everything for him without complaint. He was home instead of in the bars, so that was a nice change.

When my dad's pain lessened and his mobility improved, he took the car and headed to a local bar for a drink. He was still using crutches. Ma pleaded with him not to go, but he went anyway. One night he got home late, intoxicated, and began swinging those crutches at Ma as she huddled down in a corner. I still remember those shiny, aluminum crutches swinging horizontally through the air. After all she had done to care for him, this was her reward.

Then, a minor miracle occurred. My dad's abdomen began to swell. Medical tests revealed that he had severe cirrhosis of the liver. This forced him to stop drinking or face liver failure and the need for a transplant. He would have his abdomen tapped regularly for fluid buildup. To his credit, after all the heartache caused by the drinking, he took this liver problem to be the final sign that something had to change.

His drinking all but came to a complete stop. We never saw my dad drunk again after the liver problem was diagnosed. Dad would sneak in a half a glass of wine or half a beer but that was all. He was pleasant and this must have been a great relief to Ma.

My dad continued to scan the papers and look for work. But his large abdomen certainly gave the appearance that something was wrong and hurt his chances when it came to a face to face interview. He tried and he tried hard.

Ma worked part-time at several small jobs. Money was always a worry for her and she felt the need to contribute. On Sundays, she would make dinner for us and then drive to her job at a nursing home where she helped care for patients. She eventually had to quit this job because of the limitations she had using her left hand.

Over the next few years, my brother and sister and I moved out and off to college. These were relatively good years for my mom and dad. They didn't take any fancy vacations beyond maybe a bus trip to Tahoe for a day at the casino. They did little things like go to a baseball game or take a drive somewhere. Projects in the backyard became a joint venture between the two of them. My dad liked to experiment in the kitchen and Ma liked to brag about some special meal they cooked together. Grandma would come over and she and Ma would have tea or go out to lunch. They even took a class together at a local junior college.

In 1985, Ma was working in the yard one afternoon when she began to feel ill. She made it into the house before she collapsed and had a seizure; she was having another stroke. This again affected her left side, compounding the damage from the stroke 23 years earlier. My mom was placed in a rehabilitation hospital for a period of time. My dad worried about what further limitations she would have when she was finally home.

This stroke set Ma back with increased difficulty walking and the need to use a cane. Her left arm was now nonfunctional. Everything was slowed and required more effort. Dad stepped up and cared for her. He helped her do the things she had trouble with, like dressing and getting in and out of the bathroom. He cooked and did chores around the house. They worked together and Ma improved. Dad did a good job for my mom after this stroke.

My siblings and I were busy working and starting our own families by this time. We would visit on weekends and the two of them were getting along well together. Ma improved to the point of being able to do most everything she did before the last stroke. She was just slower and everything took more effort.

Five years later, in 1990, my dad died of lung cancer. He died ten days after being diagnosed. I believe he knew he was sick and didn't let anyone know of the pain he was in until he visited an emergency room where they made the final diagnosis. But it was too late to do anything. He must have known because this cancer had already metastasized to the bone by this time. I'm sure he just didn't want to worry Ma.

During his last two weeks, I helped my dad take a shower when he was too weak to move about alone. I remember looking up at the ceiling at one point, in sadness, knowing that he would be gone soon. I hoped so much that he was not in pain. He was a good man who stepped up when my mom needed it. One of the very last things he said to me was, "Who is going to take care of Ma?"

My appreciation for my dad would grow over the years. He was a good person who had a disease. He worked hard and did the best he could for our family. He was kind to Ma after her second stroke. There was an unspoken connection between the two of them. Ma would miss him greatly but never outwardly admit it. She processed things internally, in her own way.

Ma was now alone. She went through the grieving process by herself. She didn't have close friends. A woman from the local hospice service came to see her on a few occasions. Ma would say later she found comfort in this. On visits to see Ma, I would sit with her at the kitchen table. She'd pick at the corner of the newspaper with her right hand and say how she couldn't believe dad was gone.

How she managed those first few years after dad died I'll never know. She had lost her partner and it must have been terribly lonely. There was also the physical aspect of caring for herself all alone in that house with her disability. She never complained, never asked for help even once. Ma learned to manage.

A year or so after my dad died, we found a gun in Ma's house hidden in a paper bag, behind some furniture. When we asked her what it was for, she admitted she thought about shooting herself in the chest after dad had died. We don't know where she got the gun; we took it away. Ma was very strong and she had her own ideas about things. I think this showed the depth of her grief over my dad's passing.

My grandmother and Ma would talk every day on the phone and visit each other once or twice a week. Thank goodness for our grandmother. She never got credit for the difference she made in our lives. She died at age 92 after complications from a medical test. Ma cared for her at the end. They were very close. Ma would recall her as "Mama" later, in the years of her own confusion.

Ma lived alone for an incredible 15 years after my dad died. The boredom and loneliness she endured I can't begin to imagine. Miraculous is the only way to describe how she managed all those years. She'd give you a chuckle if you asked her how she did it. She was so unassuming and humble. She lived from one day to the next, one small step at a time.

Idleness was not something she tolerated well. She looked for small part-time jobs in the newspaper, and kept herself busy with a few little personal assistance jobs, like reading for a blind man, or shopping for a woman who, as fate would have it, was an alcoholic. Ma even bought alcohol for that woman.

She had her little "projects" in the yard as she called them. Potting a few flowers, trimming a bush, or pulling a few weeds gave her joy. This work took a long time with only one functioning arm and walking problems, but she was never deterred. She'd put on her garden hat and head out to the yard with a bucket over her stiff left arm.

I visited Ma three or four times a year with my family. She would always have the beds made and things tidied up around the house. There would be treats the kids liked in the refrigerator when we arrived. Clearly, she looked forward to our visits.

A trip to the local post office or store was quite the task for Ma. She was so proud of her ability to get into the car and start it with one hand. She managed the grocery shopping, getting gas, and other errands like banking and doctor visits all those years. The employees of these various businesses would come to know Ma and assist her as they could. They could see she needed help, but she never asked for it.

Ma would buy her clothes at the "treasure shop" when she could not sew anymore. She was so proud when she made a good find there. This was an outing for her, something that gave her pleasure. The treasure shop was the Goodwill store about two miles away. I don't believe Ma ever set foot in a department store.

Ma sent a birthday card to the three of us, on time, every year. She would simply sign the card "Ma." These cards were very important, not only because of the message in the card but because of the effort we knew it took for her to go out and get the card, address it, put the card in an envelope and seal it, all with one hand. She never missed a birthday in the 15 years she lived alone.

Each year we could see things getting harder and harder for her. Things weren't being kept up like they had been. We didn't care but it was a sign that she was slowing down. The walk down the hallway for her was painful to watch. So much effort and energy were needed just to keep from tripping over her left foot. I knew it would only get harder.

We got a brace for her but she didn't use it. She fell several times that we knew of and somehow she got up and kept moving. Ma fell in the yard on one occasion and cracked a rib or two. She never complained over the phone. We only knew this because of the pain she was still in when we arrived for a visit. Standing, walking and coughing were difficult for her. She insisted she would be fine and not to worry.

Ma's backyard was her sanctuary. She would take her digger out there and sit on a little foot stool, move some dirt around, and maybe plant a bulb or two. The fresh air and the sun on her back, she told us, felt good. Watching her, when it was windy out, you'd think she would be blown over. But that didn't bother her. She was a tightrope walker - a daredevil - in the way she manipulated herself around to get the things done she wanted to do.

Going out to get the paper in the morning took Ma ten minutes. In the cold mornings of winter, she would drag the paper up the walkway with a rake. My sister eventually planned for the paper to be placed on the porch, but that didn't happen all the time and Ma would still go out there in the early morning darkness to retrieve that paper.

Ma never used the heater in the winter, even when temperatures got down into the forties and fifties. The kids would tease that they could always see their breath in Grandma's house. Ma would simply put on an extra sweater.

During the summer, with no air conditioning, it was stiflingly hot in Ma's house. She never opened more than one window, always worried about "the weirds" climbing in. She was used to this way of living.

I would call Ma once a week to see how she was doing. Occasionally I would notice some slowness in her responses, or subtle confusion. We learned that these symptoms are often related to dehydration. I would tell her to drink more fluids, to which she would respond, "I drink water all day long." But one cup of water would last her most of the day as she took only a sip at a time. We began stocking her house with all types of liquids.

Ma had an incident or two while driving that eventually forced us to take her car keys away. This was a big blow to her. She never drove over a mile or two, but she was so proud of her ability to get out and do things for herself. Finally, she bumped into the back of someone's car in the rain one day. From then on my sister and her husband took Ma out for her errands. "Slow and methodical" was how my brother in law described Ma's way. It worked for her. She was a survivor.

There was never much in Ma's refrigerator. She ate a half sandwich for lunch and dinner, with maybe the addition of some soup or an apple and one cookie to satisfy her sweet tooth. Egg salad and peanut butter and jelly were her mainstays. Egg salad was always so laborious because of the time it took to peel an egg with one hand, but she liked it a lot.

Ma's nutrition became a concern when we noticed her losing weight. My sister would prepare meals and freeze them for Ma to heat in the microwave. Ma enjoyed these and they helped maintain her weight.

Although Ma wanted to maintain her independent living, it was becoming clearer that she was having difficulty. Her struggling manner around that house gave life meaning and purpose, even if it took her 30 minutes to change her clothes. She was on her own schedule and it didn't matter to her how long it took to do something. She didn't see the danger of the situation. Safety was becoming an issue and I knew the time was coming when a change in Ma's living situation would have to be made.

It was hard leaving Ma alone after those weekend trips, seeing her stand in the doorway waving goodbye. I worried if she would make it back to her chair without falling. It was so painful to think of her struggling alone. The time was coming when Ma would not be able to live alone and her living situation would need to change. I wanted to take her in with me and I was going to be so happy when that day came.

In November of 2004, Ma fell out in the garage and could not get back up. She spent that night sitting on a step at the back door with the temperature dropping down into the 40s. Paramedics were summoned when there was no answer to her phone the next morning. They found her cold and confused. She was hospitalized suffering from exposure and dehydration. Several weeks in a rehabilitation hospital followed.

It was clear that a decision needed to be made soon about Ma returning to her home and living alone. Remarkably, she recovered from the fall in the garage. She returned home and insisted on staying there. We knew she was out on a limb but we were not going to physically remove her from home against her will.

Home health came out to the house to provide physical therapy and follow-up care. Ma fooled them into believing she was safe to stay in her house alone. The time had come to talk to Ma about moving in with me. We could no longer let her live precariously on her own. She needed help.

As a family, we tossed around the idea of assisted living or convalescent care, but we didn't trust any of those facilities to care for her. It had been our experience that Ma's stiff limbs made the nursing staff nervous and less likely to get Ma out of bed. She needed more help than many would willingly provide. Ma had encountered a mean nurse in one rehabilitation hospital and recalled this on occasion. We weren't going to put her through any of that again. We were fearful of her dying quickly in such a facility.

The decision was made for Ma to eventually move in with me in Southern California, something I had wanted all along. I knew how to handle Ma properly. It made sense and was the most logical thing to do. I told Ma that we would have to make a change if there was another incident such as a fall or injury.

Almost an entire year passed before another fall occurred, that we were aware of, forcing the inevitable. My brother and sister and I talked and agreed it was time. Ma deserved a medal for bravery, but she could no longer live alone in her home.

THE JOURNEY

In 2005, over Labor Day weekend, Ma was brought to Southern California to live with me. I had looked forward to this day for years, knowing I would care for Ma at some point. The time had now come.

I was so excited for my sister to arrive with Ma that weekend. I couldn't sit still, waiting for the call that they were pulling into the driveway. Ma was now going to be safe and secure. The days of unhealthy cold and heat in her house were over. She would no longer be alone in that big empty house of hers, moving from one room to another at a snail's pace. Falls, injuries, and loneliness would be no more.

My relief and happiness were immeasurable. I could protect her now. She could see her grandkids' kids regularly. There would be more stimulation and she'd be able to see and experience things she hadn't before. Ma would have all the help she needed.

Nutrition for Ma would be better and she wouldn't have to work so hard for it. Even the simple things like laundry or going to the store would be taken care of for her. It was time for her to enjoy things and not live life out on a limb as she had been.

I was a divorced dad living in a two-bedroom condominium close to where my kids lived. Ma would have the master bedroom with bathroom and shower. This arrangement worked pretty well. There were even a couple of nosy neighbors across the hall who would keep Ma company at times.

Still recovering from her last fall, she needed help transferring out of her wheelchair to the toilet or bed. She could eat, and move around in her wheelchair, on her own but needed assistance with dressing, bathing and meal preparation.

I arranged for a caregiver from an agency to be with Ma while I was at work. Although Ma seemed to accept the fact that she needed help with preparation of her meals and bathroom activity, it must have been a huge adjustment for her to let go of things she was so used to doing on her own.

I thought everything was perfect until Ma began asking about going home. She would say, "I need to get home. I can't stay here forever. I have things I need to attend to." She wanted to be in her own surroundings, not mine. Even though she was close to me and her grandkids, she still felt the pull of her own home and the memories it held.

Ma's desire to go home, despite her limitations, was a bit heartbreaking. Her safety depended on having someone to look after her. While living on her own, the daily grind gave her the motivation to keep going. The chore of getting that newspaper was rewarded by the crossword puzzle she would do later. In her home, she had control over her environment and her routine. Her memories of Dad were there. Yes, we were taking her away from the things that gave her life meaning, but allowing her to live alone in her home was dangerous.

Ma had been willing to accept help given by my sister with meals and transportation for errands, but being taken away from her home was another matter. She very likely thought living with me would be a temporary situation, but she would never again see the inside of her house. This is what had to be done.

Ma knew that to go home, she would have to be able to stand and walk, at least short distances. On several occasions, at her request, I would help her try to walk. She knew that if she couldn't walk, she could never go home alone.

Reality dictated this wasn't practical or safe for her. She would try and try to stand up and move that left leg forward, but the effort was just too much. After three or four steps, with a great deal of assistance, she would have to sit down. Tough to watch, but I knew she had to see for herself that she could not do it.

I saw the look of disappointment on her face and it was striking. Her mind told her she could do it but her body said no. After a few more attempts, Ma would not walk again.

The first few years with Ma were a learning and adjustment period. We settled into the routines that worked best for both of us. I would get Ma up and dressed in the morning and feed her breakfast. Ma would then be alone for two hours before the caregiver arrived. When I got home from work, Ma would be all mine again, from six o'clock in the evening through the night, on weekdays, and all day and night on weekends and holidays.

I learned the ins and outs of meal preparation, bathing, changing clothes, diaper technology, and skin care. I learned all the things needed to care for Ma in the most efficient way possible, like how to angle her wheelchair just right at the sink, so she could brush her teeth by herself. We learned how to best get in and out of the car and the exact temperature needed for her bathwater and oatmeal. I learned that despite giving her the medications she took every morning at the same time, she still felt the need to remind me about this every day.

Different caregivers came and went during her first year and a half with me. We had to let one caregiver go because she would always play religious music. She would watch the religious channel on TV and even encourage Ma to sing. Ma was not a religious person but Ma, being the kind of person she was, didn't want to bother the caregiver during her work by asking her to change the station. My mom had the attitude that she was there for the caregiver and wanted them to be comfortable, instead of the other way around. This was the way Ma was.

My ex-wife, Nikki, would help with Ma and would even get Ma ready for bed if I couldn't be home on time. She was a nurse so she had the training. Most would say this was unusual for an ex-wife to do, but Ma was family to Nikki and that was important. I appreciated the help.

Ma seemed amused by the kids when they would come over for dinner. The stimulation may have been a bit much for her, at times, after living alone for 15 years. However, the presence of family around Ma felt good. She was part of our lives and seemed to enjoy being part of the conversations.

Caring for Ma required physical work, scheduling changes and pre-planning for outings, soccer games, and other activities. Adjustments were made for these new demands and things were going smoothly. Everything felt right.

That first year was a period of adaptation, but putting Ma to bed every night felt like the right thing for her at this point in her life. I'd give Ma a little kiss on the forehead each night and tell her to sleep well. When I left the room, I felt confirmation that bringing her into my home was the right thing to do. I could never imagine her being alone again. She was being cared for with the kindness she deserved.

The weeks, months and very soon, an entire year passed. There was always something to do and little time to take a deep breath. I was unaware that a storm was brewing on the horizon.

The first sign was a change in my temperament. I'd be patient and understanding one minute and irritable the next, for no obvious reason. I noticed this in myself but didn't connect the dots between these feelings and what was causing them. What was it that set me off so easily at times? I'd always been pretty laid back, and now I seemed rattled. The problem would eventually come into focus, but meanwhile, the ground under my compassionate self was eroding.

Into the second year with Ma, I found myself becoming increasingly repulsed by the smell of urine. I became easily irritated by such things as buttoning and unbuttoning Ma's clothing, or dealing with the uncooperative footrest of the wheelchair. Ma frequently reminded me to do things I'd done at least a thousand times before, which bothered me much more than such a simple comment ever should have.

We had arguments over the temperature of her oatmeal, if the screen door was locked or not, and whether she was going to fall while I was transferring her out of the shower. I didn't need to be reminded to give her her medication. I had taken care of it the previous 500 days. I took out my frustration on the toaster lever, or by the speed and force with which I threw Ma's diaper into the trash can.

My fuse was particularly short when I had something else to do or somewhere to go. Needing something from the store like diapers, or having to meet the kids somewhere meant the pressure was on. This is when I would triage my work or cut a corner in order to do what I had to. You can't fit three pounds of sausage in a two-pound bag. I was approaching the end of my capacity to handle what needed to be done and I was only in the second or third year.

Ma was always my primary responsibility and that never wavered. What changed was how I went about taking care of everything that needed to be done in my private life and with my work with Ma. As I realized the ramifications of caregiving upon my time, there were changes I needed to make. But I was doing too much by myself. Lack of this realization led to frustration and tension.

There were signs that should have caught my attention but I didn't realize the importance of what I was feeling. I needed a break, but instead, I forged ahead because there were no other options at the time. The seriousness of my changing effect and behavior were not on my radar screen so they never elicited a corrective action. The seriousness of my changing behavior was not on my radar screen. Therefore a corrective action was never taken. I was essentially unaware of the trouble coming for Ma and me.

When angered, I would become quiet and less communicative with Ma. I wouldn't give her a warning or an explanation of what we would be doing next. I just went ahead and did it, sometimes catching her off guard. This would happen particularly during a transfer to the bed or toilet or when moving her wheelchair. Usually, she could anticipate my moves but if I was riled up about something, I jumped the gun. This, no doubt, scared her on occasion and was one example of how my attitude affected the way I treated Ma.

Ma's desire to go home endured. From out of the blue, she would demand that a key for her house be made for her and that is was time for the renters to move. We had rented Ma's house out. The rent money was used to pay her caregiver from the agency.

The following is a transcript of a handwritten letter my mom wrote to my sister in 2008, two and a half years since her arrival in my home.

Patricia,

I am growing more and more homesick all the time and I want to go home before the house is sold. Once that happens it is gone for good

I am in the wrong place when I can't go to the toilet when I have to, but in my house, I could. Another thing is not being able to walk more. I know what I need but John is too controlling to let me have it. (A cane)

John is also angry all the time and very uptight. He can throw something or bang something. If I'm too slow moving my bad leg or arm, I'm the one who will get pushed, pulled or shook.

John has done a lot for me here with meals, showers, exercise, but it is all too much for him and me.

The people renting the house will just have to rent another house. Start thinking about grandma's house, sell or rent, but empty is bad. Call me after Julie leaves at noon.

Ma

This letter incensed me when I eventually read it. Never was Ma pushed, pulled, or shook. She was difficult to move and I always did my best to prevent injury to her and myself. This criticism was the type of thing that chewed into my desire to continue caregiving. Every negative comment or judgment, about how something was being done, would alienate me just a bit more from my caregiving duty.

At this point, Ma had been with me for only two and a half years. Seven and a half more years were to come. Fortunately, some adaptation did occur to the idiosyncrasies of caregiving during the middle years. The button thing didn't bother me anymore, nor did the footrest of the wheelchair or the request for medication. Thank God for the ability to adapt. Still, there was a long way to go. I would ask myself every Labor Day weekend how many more years there would be.

Ma came along on small trips I would take with the kids. A few of their friends would usually go with us. Ma was annoyed by the food fights, childish humor and roughhousing that were part of kids being kids. Even though the kids made her nervous, it was nice to have her along with us. She experienced things she wouldn't have otherwise, and she could get away from the house for a few days.

When visitors came by they would always remark what a sweet person Ma was. She was basically a shy person, but she took an interest in anyone who would sit and talk with her. Visitors seemed to make Ma happy and people responded to her in a positive way.

Doctor's appointments were few and far between because Ma was very healthy. She rarely even got a cold, and she refused the flu shot. The doctor would get a kick out of Ma's frank responses to questions. Ma drank cranberry juice every morning and regularly throughout the day. She suffered very few bladder infections through the years, even though she wore a diaper all day. I attributed this to the cranberry juice.

Occasionally Ma would become somewhat dehydrated. She would seem slower, more tired, frequently more confused. I could tell by the weight of her diaper in the morning if she wasn't getting enough fluid. Less urine output meant the need for more input. If her diaper did not feel a certain weight, I knew we had to increase her fluids, and she would respond quickly to this.

Ma's blood pressure was taken every day and recorded. She monitored these recordings herself, even when there was little change from day to day. Ma's few medications were easy for me to get, as her pharmacy was just across the parking lot from my work. Most caregivers don't have the luxury of such convenience when filling prescriptions and the task can be a source of distress. We maintained organization of Ma's medications but she knew if ever we missed a pill. She took great interest in any lab work and wanted the reports read to her in full.

Ma always ate well, but very slowly. We would all be done eating and Ma would be only halfway through her meal. She was quite happy being the last person sitting at the table. She could finish eating in peace.

We had a system if Ma needed something in the middle of the night. Her bed was against the wall in her room which adjoined my room. She would give a tap on the wall with her right hand which I could easily hear. When she did knock, it was usually for reasons related to seeing things in her room that weren't there. I would go into her room occasionally, in the middle of the night, just to check on her and I'd find her awake. She may have had some fear of the dark. We used a night light and tried various things to help her sleep. None of these worked well but eventually, the episodes of sleeplessness passed.

I could leave Ma alone for periods of time in the beginning. If she had water available, she was more than willing to sit and watch TV. She could propel her wheelchair around if need be. She was unable to get out of her chair on her own but she could get to a window or a book or a cookie by propelling the wheelchair with her right arm and leg.

One day she was alone and I came home to find her on the floor. After the caregiver left, she fell while attempting to stand by herself. I thought we had discouraged this activity, but apparently not enough. She cracked her pelvis and had to spend a month in a rehabilitation hospital. I had thought about restraining Ma in the wheelchair, especially when Ma's talk or actions indicated she might try to get up out of her chair, but I never did. I felt that having something around her might just challenge her to get out of her chair all the more.

I had put the condominium up for sale and it sold just before Ma's fall. I found a house and was able to move in just as Ma was to be discharged from the rehabilitation hospital. The new house was handicapped accessible and worked out nicely for Ma. We now had a steady caregiver from an agency named Julie. At $17.50 per hour, it was expensive but worth the peace of mind.

I worked an average of 50 hours a week. I left the house at 8 in the morning and returned home about 6 in the evening. Before I left for work I would get Ma up and fix her breakfast. The caregiver came about an hour after I left and prepared lunch and dinner for Ma. Julie's duties also included Ma's laundry, dishes after meals and some light housework like sweeping or vacuuming. She also made sure Ma received fluids and snacks throughout the day.

Ma did not trust anyone but me to give her a shower. She was confident in how I moved her onto the shower chair. Ma was deathly afraid of slipping and falling during this activity and she felt the most secure when I did it for her. It would have been nice if the caregiver could have done this occasionally because I never looked forward to it. Ma and I would regularly have conflict over the temperature of the water. But when we were done, Ma would say, "Well, ya did it again." That was her way of saying thank you. We both had a sense of accomplishment when Ma felt refreshed after her shower.

We adjusted the caregiver's hours based on need. We attempted a split shift at one point, having Julie work two hours in the morning and return for three hours in the afternoon. When Julie was sick, the agency sent out a replacement. The replacements were very nice and they all got a kick out of Ma and her sweet disposition. But Ma's favorite was Julie.

Even though they had become friends I got the feeling, at one point, that Julie wasn't doing all that could be done for Ma in terms of stimulation. I felt she was spending too much time just watching TV. When I'd ask Ma about what Julie did, she would compliment her, defend her, and say she was doing everything she needed to be doing.

Nevertheless, I set out a schedule of activities for Julie to do with Ma. They would play Bingo or word games every morning before lunch. They would go outside for fresh air at least once a day, weather permitting. The radio would be used for news or some entertainment in the afternoon. I didn't want the TV to be the sole source of stimulation.

Julie seemed to see what I was trying to accomplish and was cooperative with the routine. This lasted a couple of years. Ma was doing well. She was healthy and doing well.

Ma read books, mainly biographies, and a lot of them. She was a Hollywood trivia buff and could recall the names of actresses and actors so well. People loved having a conversation with her regarding the old-time movies. Turner Classic Movies was Ma's favorite TV channel and she perked up whenever one of her old favorites aired.

Attempts were made to have her go to an adult day care center for some socialization. Ma declined, stating she didn't want the trouble and preferred just to stay home. I wish I had been more persuasive about this at the time. A change of scenery and a conversation with others would have been good for Ma.

For reasons unknown to me, I never considered Ma going to adult day care as respite care for myself. I was wrapped up in Ma's daily care and didn't appreciate how I was being affected and changed. I couldn't see this as a small, but obvious, potential solution to a problem because I hadn't yet identified the problem. My drum was too tight but I didn't recognize the need to fix it.

I also didn't recognize the strain that caregiving imposed on my relationships with just about everyone. This included work, where people would comment that I often looked tired or stressed. Some found me to be standoffish at times. My work required that I talk to people all day. When I got home I needed to care for Ma. I had no interest in befriending any of the neighbors or listening to their small talk.

My relationship with Darlene was most certainly affected by caregiving because there didn't seem to be enough of me to go around. There were expectations of me to attend certain functions, but often I was simply too tired to be out late at night. That meant having to make arrangements for someone to watch Ma, which Darlene often took care of. However, I did not want to impose on others. I'd rather just stay home or, if I did go out, be able to leave in time to be home again when I was needed there.

I cannot blame Darlene for wanting to have a real relationship with all its normal benefits. She hung in there at times when I'm sure there was something she'd rather be doing than spending time at my house with Ma. My time constraints meant that she had to sacrifice a great deal to be with me.

Darlene was very generous and loving toward Ma. She doted over Ma in a way that made her feel special and cared for. This was a great assist to me. I was admittedly short on some of the softer subtleties of what makes a woman feel like a woman. Ma had simple needs but the way Darlene combed her hair made her feel good, and I could never quite do it the same way.

While Darlene was doing nice things for Ma, I was antagonized by the feeling that she did the easy work or the feel-good stuff while she knew very little of what went on behind the scenes with Ma's care. Instead of being thankful for the help she gave, I showed virtually no appreciation for what she did. I couldn't even be happy for Ma that nice things were being done for her. In hindsight, it is obvious how wrong I was.

One morning Julie's legs got entangled with Ma's leg as she was attempting to transfer her. This resulted in a fractured lower leg on Ma's left side. Ma was placed back in the rehabilitation hospital for about a month. This was a nice break for me, no pun intended. Life was easier with no set schedules. I could stay out later and possibly be a better boyfriend. There was enjoyment in the ability to come and go without worry about leaving Ma alone.

Ma's left leg was the same one affected by her stroke and not used heavily during transfers, so this injury didn't decrease Ma's mobility too much. The therapy staff worked with Ma on standing and walking. I was leery of this because I didn't want Ma to get any ideas that she would be walking when she returned home. Just the idea of walking could lead Ma to try to get up by herself when alone and potentially cause a major injury with a fall.

Ma tended to think she could still do things she couldn't. Her insight and awareness regarding safety were impaired due to the strokes. If there had been a freeway out front, she would have walked across it to see the neighbor. We didn't want to encourage her.

Ma developed an ulcer on her heel while in the rehabilitation hospital. Home health came out to the house every day for the next six months attending to that wound. I think the benefit of these visits for Ma was more for social stimulation than it was for wound healing. I didn't mind. Another human being for Ma to talk to was a good thing.

Ma continued to believe she could go home and live alone. "I've got to go home," she would say with all seriousness. There were no additional letters written by Ma and, her going home again wasn't even a remote possibility. Reasoning with Ma about this was difficult. In her mind, she was being kept away from her home. She felt she still had the ability to function there with some assistance. She would ask about taking Julie with her and say that she had work to do at home. These pleas to go home faded over the years and that, by itself, was sad to witness.

I can't imagine the boredom Ma must have felt, missing the activities she previously enjoyed at her house. Her "projects" were what had kept her going. Now everything was being done for her. Day after day, week after week, month after month Ma's routine was the same: suffocating idleness. I'd come home from work and find her rolling aimlessly around the house in her wheelchair or asleep with her head in a book.

Ma was an animal lover. She took care of dogs, cats, rabbits, mice and a tortoise through the years. These animals lived long lives because of the care Ma gave them, minus the tortoise who disappeared in a storm one night. Ma's love for the simple tasks of caring for her animals and the labor she put into her yard, even with her physical handicap, would create great respect for Ma in anyone who witnessed these things. She was truly remarkable.

I had a dog during Ma's stay with me. Her name, given to her by a previous owner, was Gongju. Ma didn't care for that name and preferred to call her "Short Stuff" instead. One of the little tasks Ma gave herself to do during the day was making sure there was water in Short Stuff's bowl. Several times a day Ma would let her out in the yard to do her business. Short Stuff knew exactly where walk so as not to get run over by Ma's wheelchair in the process.

I can't count all the times I saw Ma reach down with her right hand to give that dog a little pat on the top of the head. Short Stuff would give Ma a quick lick on her hand and then be off, sniffing around the bottom of Ma's wheelchair for food she may have dropped. Having Short Stuff was a small thing, but she meant a lot to Ma and was good for her.

Three or four years into Ma's stay with me, I was forced to take a 10% pay cut at work. Since there were some expenses I had to cover in caring for Ma, this was an additional stress on me. I felt the need to ask my brother and sister for financial assistance. They were both very cooperative and agreed to send me a certain amount of money every month. This greatly relieved the financial portion of my stress, but many caregivers do not have such support.

I was grateful for this help from my brother and sister but as time went on, I began to feel entitled to the money. I appreciated the financial contribution from my brother and sister but I was the one giving up my freedom, enduring the restrictions on my life that came with the duty of caring for Ma. There was no compensation for that.

I'm not placing blame on anyone in this matter. This is just the way it was. My sister lived 400 miles away and my brother 2000 miles away. Both had jobs and their own families., I was the most qualified to care for Ma and did not expect physical help from my brother or sister. This was my job, my responsibility. But the loss of my freedom, on top of my caregiving work, made it easy to rationalize accepting that money from them.

Birthdays and holidays were particularly enjoyable for both Ma and me. Extra effort was put into sprucing Ma up for these occasions. She would have a shower. My daughter may have trimmed and painted her nails. Darlene would comb her hair extra nice. Ma would pick out her clothes to wear that day. I always tried to make it a special event for her.

Ma was in the presence of family who gave her love and attention. She perked up and would engage in conversations. There was a buzz in the air that cut into the doldrums of the daily routine. I was happy to see Ma involved; this was one of the reasons I wanted her to be with me in the first place. Later at night, when the day was over and I was getting her ready for bed, I'd always say what a nice day it had been. She would agree with a soft little smile.

As the time passed, Ma seemed to become unmoved by the holidays and presence of family. Her spike in alertness and level of socialization shrank. She would often be left alone after the hellos and would put her head down to rest. She was probably still listening, just not participating like she had previously. The interest she had shown in others was replaced by sleeping, as the activity continued around her.

Darlene had a good idea. We purchased a recliner so Ma wouldn't have to take naps in her wheelchair. This encouraged her to sleep even more during the day, but at least she seemed comfortable. This recliner would become the axis of her world during daytime hours.

When Ma's eyesight began to deteriorate, it became harder for her to read. We attempted new glasses but they didn't seem to work well and Ma would try to read without them. Gradually, Ma did fewer puzzles and read fewer books. This had been a great source of entertainment for her. It was sad to see it slide away. Mind activity and stimulation were replaced by watching TV and sleeping more during the day.

The visual changes marked a point of definite decline. When Julie, the caregiver, tried to read to Ma or help her do a crossword puzzle, her attention would fade quickly. These activities came to an end. The puzzle books and biographies that Ma had spent hours on every day were stored away and never used again.

At one point, Ma had to have her top teeth removed and a denture made. She was happy with the denture, and proudly showed off her new smile for all to see. For me, there were added duties each day of gluing it in before meals and cleaning it after. Ma really wanted to have good success with that denture, but there always seemed to be a problem with its fit and adhesion. It would come loose with warm fluids and this would interfere with her eating. We tended to use the denture less and less. Ma seemed to get by just as easily without it but we tried to use it anyway.

Then one day the denture fell out of Ma's mouth onto the floor and she ran over it with her wheelchair. It was cracked and we never used it again. We changed Ma's diet to softer (however less satisfying and nutritious) food. She did the best she could to chew, always slow and easy.

The loss of the denture and subsequent change in diet affected Ma's vitality. Ma drank fluid more often. She went through cases of Ensure. We did the best we could to encourage Ma to eat and she had her good days and bad days. I would get reports that Ma would eat 80 to 90 percent of her food one day and 30 percent or so the next.

Watching Ma struggle with her food was heartbreaking. Right before our eyes, we saw her fail at something she had done all her life. It was sad to see the look of dismay on her face when she would work so hard to get a bite of food up to her mouth only to have it fall into her lap. Half of her food would end up on the floor. She was always very skilled with the use of her right hand. Now the spoon wasn't going where she wanted.

For Ma to get enough out of each meal, we began to feed her. This increased my time requirement for caregiving and lessened my time for my own things. I found myself becoming increasingly frustrated with meal times. Feeding was never without a mess. The denture issues, the additional help needed to feed Ma, and the increased difficulty communicating with Ma all added to the demands of feeding time.

In certain instances, I found myself wanting to minimize my time with Ma. I would usually get Ma up around 9:30 in the morning on Saturday and Sunday. This became closer to 10:00 or even 10:30 on some weekends, if I was involved in something else. I would look for things to do, just to delay the inevitable. The thought of going into Ma's room to get her up for Saturdays became daunting. This was especially true if I had a long week at work. Dealing with the diaper, changing clothes, and the feeding challenges all seemed as if I had done them only an hour ago, when it was actually the night before, twelve hours earlier.

On a typical Saturday or Sunday around noon I would position Ma in her recliner in front of the TV. This allowed me to do the things I needed to do, like some yard work or going to the store. Every thirty minutes or so I would come in and check on her. After giving her a sip or two of fluid, I'd ask if she was ok and she always said, "Yes."

Around one o'clock I would try to feed Ma some lunch. Her favorite was a peanut butter and jelly sandwich and a glass of milk. In the beginning, she could eat this all on her own. Later, when she began to have trouble manipulating the sandwich with her hand, half of it would end up in her lap or on the floor. This meant I'd have to stay with her during lunch to feed her, at prime time on Saturdays and Sundays, when I felt I needed to be doing other things.

This would push me out of whack when I couldn't do what I wanted to do, when I wanted to do it. I didn't have control. The situation was controlling me. I had to do for Ma what needed to be done. If I hadn't been so wound up, I would have realized that what I was bent on doing didn't absolutely need to be done right then. I should have just picked a better time when there wouldn't be an interruption. After all, Ma did come first. It sounds simple but I didn't see it that way at the time.

If she had to go to the bathroom I would grind my teeth some, wash my hands, and take her to the bathroom. I let this interruption get to me much too easily at times. I am sure Ma disliked having to ask me to take her to the bathroom. She asked only when she had to go and would do so reluctantly. She wished she could do this alone and not bother me. Ma was aware.

My verbal interaction with Ma was minimal some days since my moods varied between cheerful and testy. I was talkative and encouraging with Ma one day then, the next, I would be quiet and mechanical with her care. In this regard, I don't think outside influences in my life affected me as much as the job of caregiving itself.

I didn't have the energy or motivation to do more than what was absolutely needed for Ma some days. If the day started off bad, with interruptions and delays, my negative mood tended to linger throughout the day. I should have had the ability to step back and make a better decision about how to do things. Trying to do too much at one time and overreacting to the smallest inconvenience made things worse.

About six years into the care of Ma we lost her caregiver Julie. She had to move to another area for family reasons. I decided to change agencies at the time and did so knowing we would never find another Julie.

One day, just after the new agency started, I came home from the store and found Ma on the floor. The new agency was not working that day. Ma's left non-functional arm was caught underneath her. As I sat her back in her chair, she winced in pain, with the movement of her left arm. I determined it was not seriously injured because it was movable and not seriously painful. The next day a bruise appeared on the outside of her elbow, but she seemed to be fine without any complaints.

The following day, the caregiver noticed the bruise, was concerned, and called her supervisor. This supervisor overreacted and had Ma transferred via ambulance to the closest hospital where an x-ray showed a small chip fracture. I picked Ma up at the hospital after work. There was no treatment suggested for the arm beside support, and Ma required no medication. This was her nonfunctional left arm and it would heal in time.

I subsequently fired that home health agency for what I felt was an overreaction to a minor incident. I went through another agency or two before deciding on hiring a caregiver privately. However, the agency that was replaced apparently contacted a county social worker who came to the house for "visits" on several occasions. Of course, they were checking up on me to assure there was no abuse occurring. Ma answered all their questions which seemed to satisfy them and the visits stopped.

This experience propelled me further down the line of wanting something different for myself. It was insulting, almost surreal, to have someone come into my home to see if things were being done properly. I had chosen to do this and I was working hard to assure Ma's safety. Now I was under watch for something so minor that Ma had forgotten about it a day or two after it occurred. Who needed this? I wanted it to be over.

71

We had Ma participate in the process of picking a new caregiver. Applicants were interviewed and we hit the jackpot. The new caregiver was named Paula. She would come to love Ma. Paula was very attentive and communicated with me regularly about anything out of the ordinary with Ma. It was such a relief to have someone like Paula caring for Ma. My attentiveness and patience were continuing to erode and we were lucky to find Paula.

My relationship with Ma, the mother-son relationship, was suffering as the years went by. This was the most unfortunate byproduct of the caregiving process. I cannot say enough about how surprising and discouraging this was. It affected my ability to be tolerant and compassionate with Ma. If I had spent five minutes a day with Ma, as her son, just sitting and talking about nothing in particular, I would have been a better caregiver.

Instead, I often found it difficult to be home all the time with Ma. I would get antsy and feel the need to get out of there, even if it were just to get a coffee or soda. The recliner became the method of security I needed to leave Ma alone. It allowed me to take advantage of Ma's immobility. Putting Ma in the recliner meant I could leave her alone and not worry she would fall or stray into a corner. I could go to the movies or out to dinner or see the kids. Leaving her alone like this may not have been the right thing to do, but I needed it to provide some breathing space in my life.

Many caregivers do not have this little bit of freedom I enjoyed because of Ma's immobility. Some caregivers cannot go into the next room without fear of leaving their family member at risk for a disaster. Much like taking care of a young child, they are tethered to the person in their charge. My mom could not stand up or walk and I used this to my advantage.

I always tried to limit my time away and felt the pressure to get home. When I was with others, they never knew how I felt until they would push it, by suggesting we go do something else. Then I would have to stand up and say "Hey, I have something I need to tend to, don't you remember?" It always made me angry to have to remind people.

One night I went to the movies with Darlene and left Ma home in her recliner in front of the TV. The movie ended about 9 pm, the time I would normally be getting Ma ready for bed. We were hungry after the movie and I wanted to get some takeout so I could get home for Ma. When Darlene wanted to go somewhere for a sit-down dinner in a restaurant, it created a rift between us. I felt the pressure to get home and thought she should have understood that without me having to explain, especially since I'd known her for 8 years.

Darlene did accommodate my schedule with Ma on so many occasions and I am thankful for that. Those times when she would forget were innocent but still very frustrating for me. This is an example of the added stress that can exist in the caregiver's world. It is not easy to be the companion of a caregiver. Your time together is limited and you don't have the freedom other couples enjoy.

I always had Ma on the back of my mind. Did I push the limits beyond what I should have in terms of leaving Ma alone at times? Yes, I did. I was always aware of her needs but that's no excuse or justification for leaving her alone. I would explain where we were going and when we would be home. Every time I left the house, the ever-present worry that she would fall out of the chair went with me. It was a calculated risk that I took because I would have gone crazy without the occasional little break to go out to dinner or a movie.

I took Ma wherever I could but often she would decline to go. I remember wanting to take her to the beach for a ride down the pier in her wheelchair. How great it would be for her to feel the nice, cool ocean air on her face. It took some doing but I finally convinced her to go one Saturday. When we got to the pier, she was deathly afraid of falling into the water. Never mind we were rolling her down the middle of the 30-foot-wide pier. She was a nervous wreck and it wasn't worth the effort to try to convince her it was safe. She did, however, enjoy a nice chocolate shake on the way home.

Outings such as going out to dinner with the kids happened less and less frequently. It was harder to get Ma in and out of the car. She wouldn't eat very well and to deal with the profuse drooling at times was a chore. I even doubted that Ma was having fun anymore on these occasions.

On a Sunday evening in March of 2015, Ma suffered what we believe was a TIA or trans-ischemic attack while she was sitting in her recliner. Darlene and I were home with her at the time. Ma's eyes turned gray and her responsiveness suddenly changed. Her body became limp. She would not answer questions and appeared listless.

This blankness and odd eye color passed within 30 minutes and it was very scary. I'd never seen anything like this before. Ma was always a rock and to see her so vulnerable, to whatever was going on in her head, was frightening.

At one point during this episode, Ma commented to Darlene "This is the end of life." We were taken aback by this comment. She knew. She knew what was happening to her.

There had been a slow decline of Ma's abilities but this was the first major event that highlighted how frail Ma was becoming. She was such a fixture, an endurable figure who took many hits and yet survived. How could it be now that Ma may be taking a definitive slide toward the end of life?

Up to this point, there had been much good in the care of Ma. I was a not a tyrant despite the rough patches and periods of heightened stress and tension. This account is a summary of ten years. Most of it was good. But I was fatigued and burned out. I didn't acknowledge the signs that things were getting the best of me. My level of stress at times affected the way I thought and acted, making it hard to be loving and compassionate.

There were days when I surprised myself with how positive, patient, and sociable I was with Ma. I wished I could have remained like this all the time, but the bottom would fall out. I was overextended.

The peaks and valleys of my ability to be a compassionate caregiver were in close succession. This reality is, to this day, hard to accept. I was running out of gas, sputtering along, with road still ahead of me.

I found the negative progression of my disposition over the ten years of caring for Ma to be remarkable. The decline from an upbeat, enthusiastic, attentive and protective person I once was to the exhausted, indifferent, callous person I became is difficult to accept.

There were days when I surprised myself with how positive, patient and sociable I was with Ma. That is the way it should have been all the time. But I was tired and my temperament would flip the other direction way too easily. The peaks and valleys of my ability to be a compassionate caregiver were surprising. I was running out of gas with a long road still ahead of me.

My perspective and attitude were outside the boundary of where they should have been in the care for Ma, especially over the last couple years. This should have never happened. I was pressed up against the problem and unable to see the whole picture. Like tunneling through a mountain and unable to turn around, I strived to see light at the end. I was committed to seeing this through, but I had no method of dealing with the stress.

I would often think about when and how Ma would eventually go and I had thoughts of it finally being over. She could be free of boredom, declining abilities and lack of control and I could be free to live my life. The end was coming. It would be nothing like what I wanted for Ma and me.

75

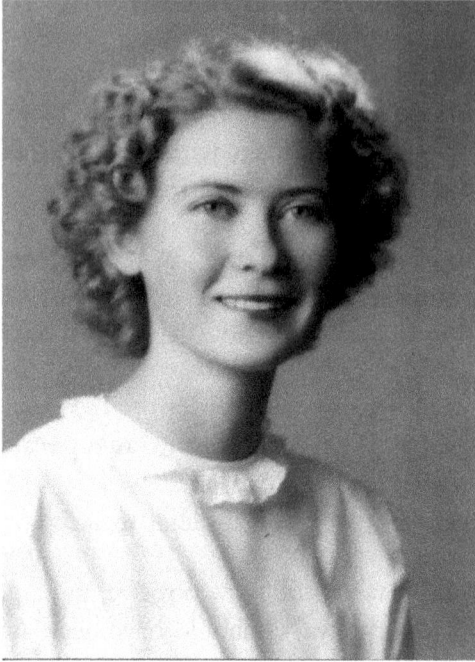

1.

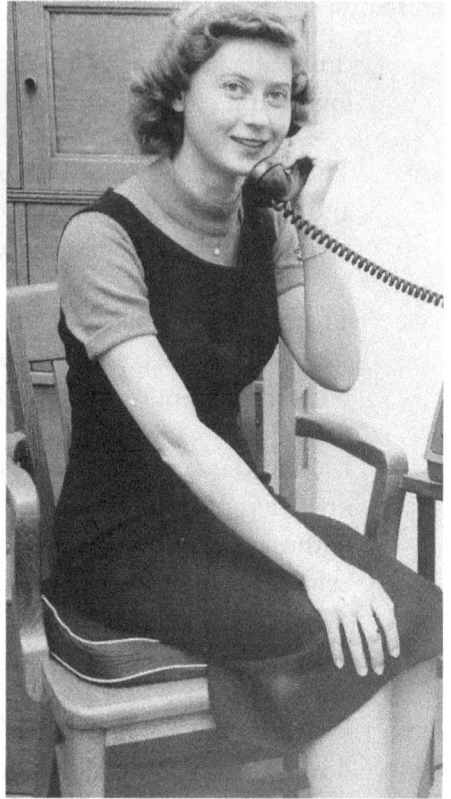

2.

1. High school picture of Ma. She's about 17 years old.
2. My mom was 27 or so here. She had a job with the phone company.
3. Picture of a picnic in 1956 where my Mom and Dad met each other for the very first time. Dad, at the right looking down. Ma in sleeveless dress, glasses, looking over her right shoulder.

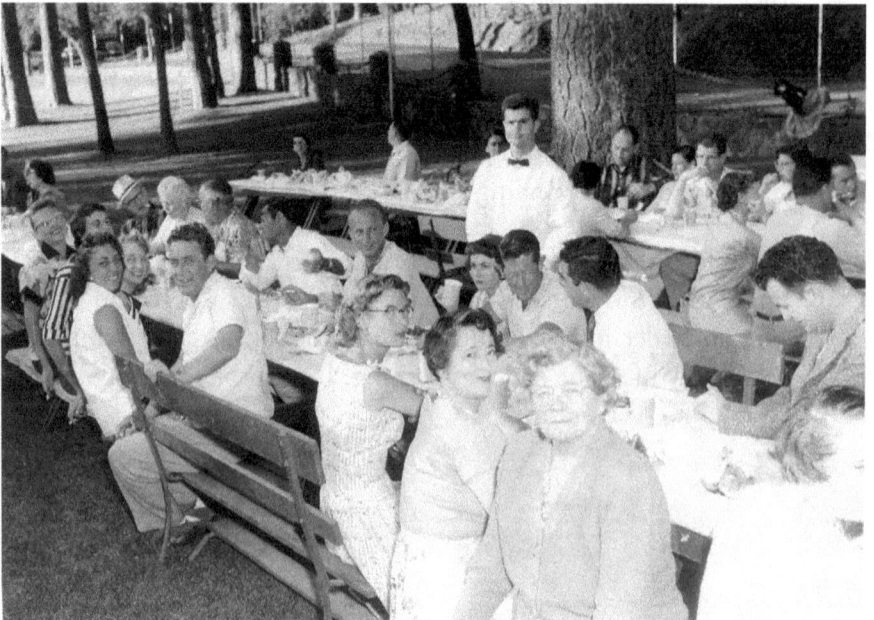

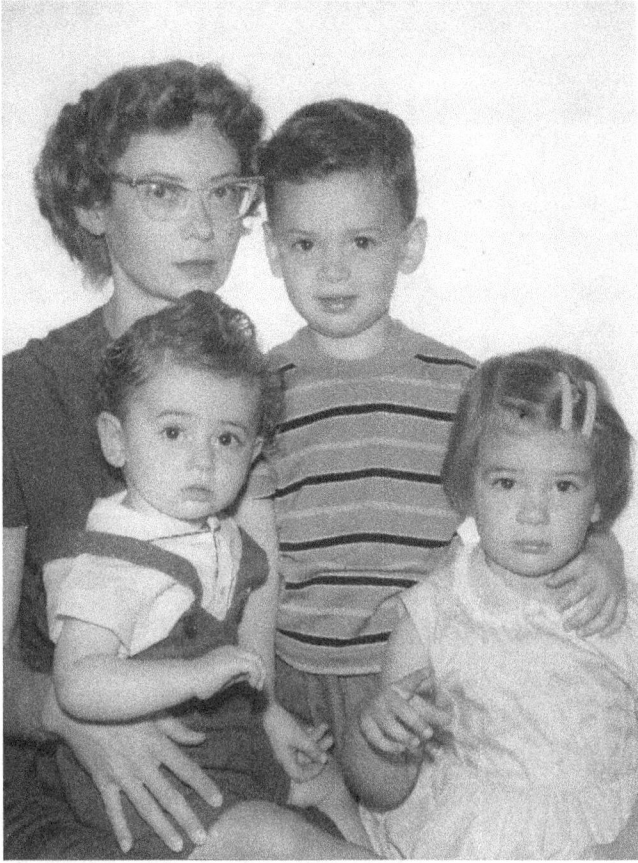

4. A picture of Ma and her three children just prior to her first stroke.
5. These are my grandparents on my mom's side. They were a huge help to us, and influence on us, at this young age.
6. One of the trips my mom would take us on. This one to the Russian River in Northern California. My brother and sister are seated next to Ma.

5.

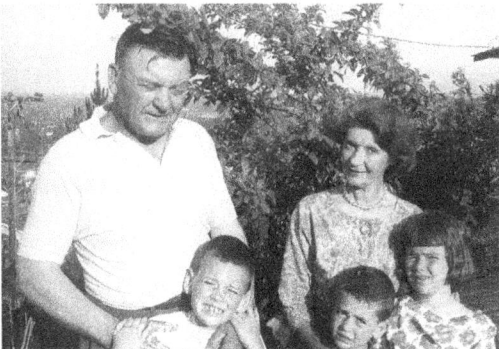

6.

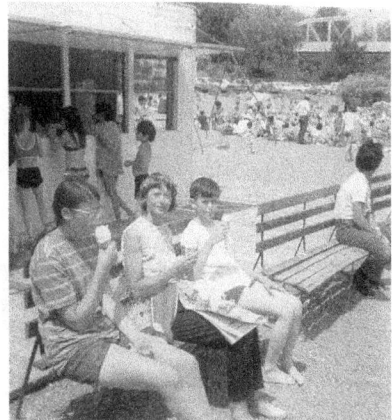

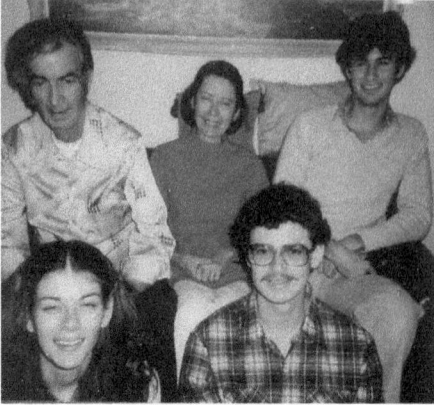

7.

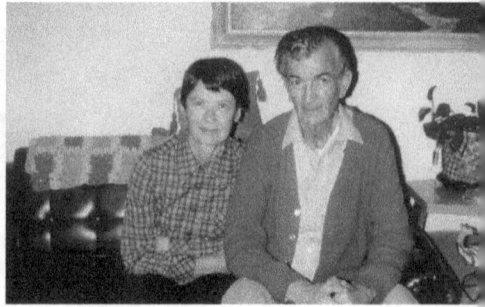

8.

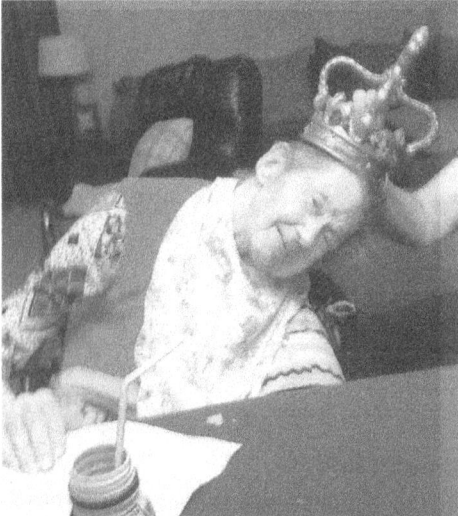

9.

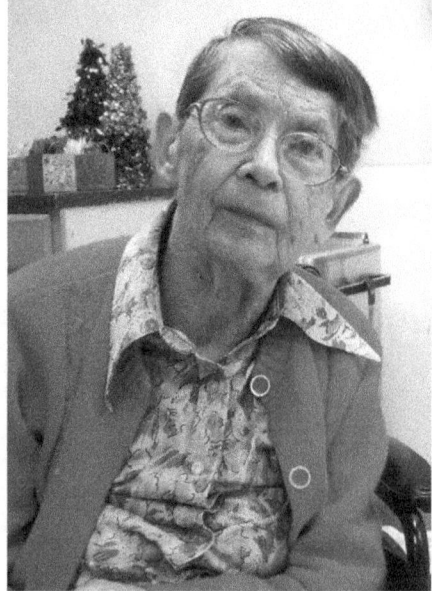

10.

7. The family in the college years for my brother, sister, and I.

8. My mom and dad in the good years, not too long before my mom's second stroke.

9. We always tried to make mom feel like a queen.

10. My mom early on in her stay with me at a Christmas party.

11. Ma with three of her grandchildren, my children.

11.

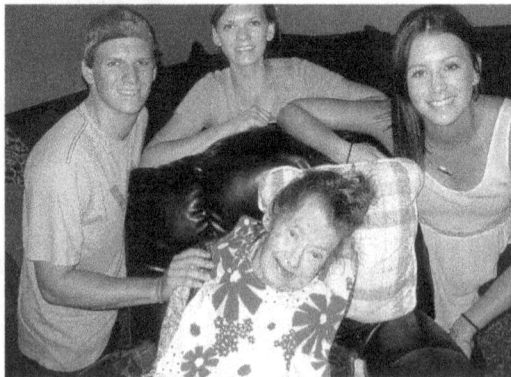

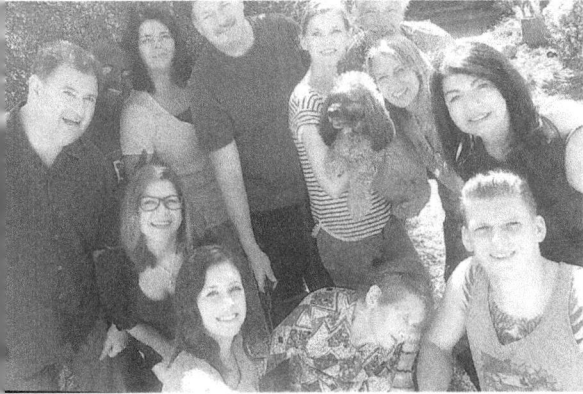

12.

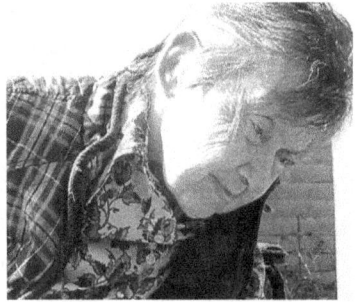

13.

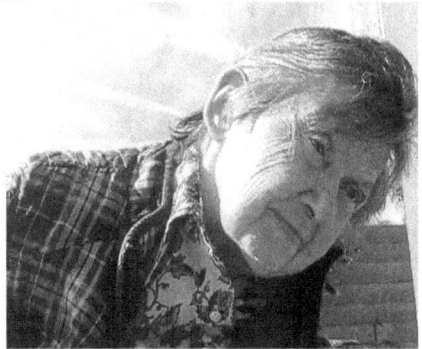

14.

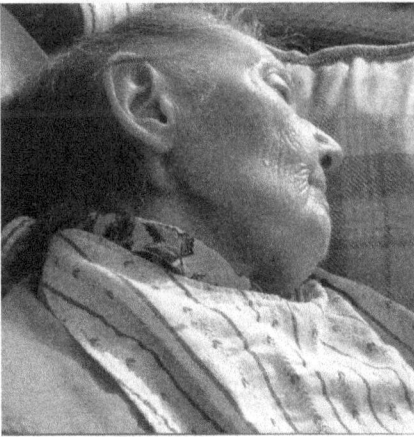

15.

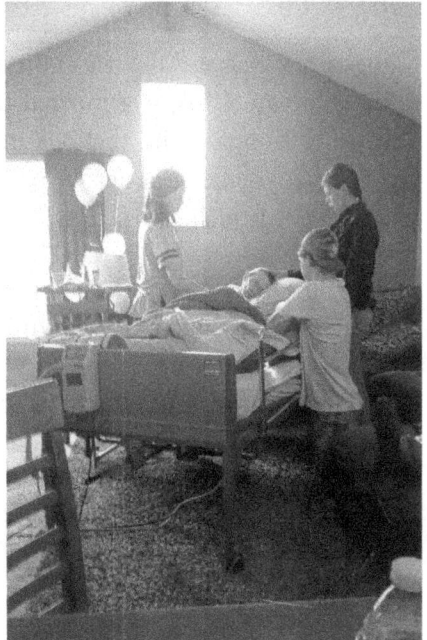

16.

12. A selfie of the entire family seven months or so prior to Ma's death.

13. A glimpse of Ma during her final six months.

14. And another.

15. Ma during the last 2 or 3 months in her recliner, resting.

16. Grandchildren at Ma's bedside just days prior to her passing.

THE LAST EIGHT MONTHS

Ma's period of altered consciousness was a real shaker for me. Yes, there was a decline in her abilities, but never was there such an incident that framed the fact that Ma could be approaching death. This incident was out of character. She was such a survivor and now it seemed this was threatened.

Previous conflicting feelings had existed within me causing unease and guilt. I feared Ma's death, but I craved the relief that would come with it. She would be free of the boredom and demise of her physical and mental abilities. I could have my life back. The realization of this suddenly became closer.

I was always hesitant to express the feelings of frustration, and the wanting for this work to be done with. Never did I want to sound like I was complaining. I didn't want to appear weak or disappoint those who had faith in my caring for Ma. I always tried to put on a good face. I pretended I was fine and all was good. In reality, I was sputtering along, but what purpose would it serve to express this?

For some reason, the thought suddenly occurred to me to write things down. I began a journal that Sunday night after Ma's "turn." Putting thoughts and feelings down on paper and closing the book seemed to make it easier to put them to bed. Regretfully, I should have started this journal long before this point.

Pinning down my exact feeling was difficult if I depended solely on thoughts. Writing things down helped me express what I was feeling and release pent-up emotion. I had to write fast or the thought would leave my head almost as soon as they arrived.

I felt my compassion was wearing thin. Quite surely Ma detected this, even through her decreased senses. Was this natural human behavior for me to be like this, something that couldn't be avoided? An inevitable slippery slope of declining caregiving ability? Or was I simply out of gas?

The point of sharing this journal is to feel the flow of emotion over Ma's last eight months of life. I was never angry with Ma. I was angry with the impact caregiving had on my life. Ma deserved the best of care but I was unable to provide this after ten years of trying to manage everything myself. None of it seemed fair, almost like some cruel right of passage was the end Ma's life.

Complete honesty is expressed here or else this is worthless fiction. The following is verbatim from my journal. This begins in March of 2015 on a Sunday night.

The following is verbatim from my journal. This begins in March of 2015 on a Sunday night.

Suddenly she is gone. Where did she go? That person I feel frustrated and burned out caring for is gone. I want her back, if only just for a moment so I can say what I want to say but never took the time to. Please come back Ma. You've done it before.

She asked me for the first time, 'Who are you?

I feel guilty about the aggravation I have felt. I don't know how much of this surfaced. I feel she sensed it. I'm sure she felt it and knew. How much more does she know? Does she hear the sidebar conversations and say to herself, 'Am I really that bad?' What fear that must cause in her. Does she wonder if she will be cared for properly? Terrible to think she may feel this way. I can't tell what is going on inside of her head. Her mind is failing and she cannot express what she wants to.

I requested Hospice services from Ma's doctor. I wanted to be prepared for anything that could happen. A nurse began coming twice a week and there was a social worker and clergy person who came about once a month. This was an excellent service. Paula was still her very caring self, but the extra attention Ma received was comforting. Later a nurse's aide came to give Ma a bed bath. What a treat that was for both me and Ma.

Ma was down for about a week following this TIA (trans-ischemic attack). She never returned to her prior level of alertness. She slept more and ate less. Talking became infrequent as she had trouble completing full sentences. This appeared to frustrate her. With all the physical and mental changes, she knew she was deteriorating. How brave she was.

This incident restored my sense of compassion for Ma. This seemed to jolt me back in line in terms of being attentive and comforting for Ma. But the effect would be temporary, as you will see.

I've taken care of her, but how have I done? Now she thinks I'm trying to hurt her. The past 10 years changing diapers, staying home rather than getting out, preparing food while thinking I was sacrificing my life. Sounds selfish of me.

Where did it change from the right thing to do for your mother to work, a chore? I see the end is in sight. There is some relief there, but it's not really what I want. I don't want to face it. It is sad.

Why did she have to struggle with this stroke all of her life? What was the reason? It seems cruel, like a punishment. She has to know she has done a great job. Tell her this before it is too late.

Somewhere, I've lost my relationship with her as my mother. It's different. It's not the same and feels as if something has been lost. If I could be with her for some other reason than changing her clothes or wiping food from her mouth, maybe it could be different. The energy needed to simply sit with her and talk about nothing and be happy with that is gone. My next interaction with her will be cleaning her in the bathroom. That takes a lot of energy. I can't afford to sit and be her son for 10 minutes.

How sad this way of thinking was and another symptom that I was on a path I shouldn't have been. I should have never let the job of caregiving come first before my relationship with her. I should have prevented this.

Ma lets us feed her with no resistance. Is that part of giving up? She now depends on us for her nourishment. She drools profusely from the left side of her mouth making a mess of her clothing. Hopefully she knows nothing of this.

I don't understand my periods of frustration. They happen usually at night, sometimes when her arm or leg won't cooperate. Other times for no reason at all. When the 9 to 10 minutes where I have to put my mind somewhere else becomes 12 to 13 minutes, that's when it hits. That's not a lot, but it feels like an eternity.

That I may have expressed anger or impatience with Ma and she sensed my feelings causes me guilt. I should have been ready for those times when she needed me more than others. If had taken more consistent breaks and time to decompress myself I would have been better able to patiently deal with an inconvenience or delay in our routine.

Why didn't I take the time to talk to her all those nights, during changing times? Now time is short. I want some of it back.

Taking her out of the house used to be a good thing. Getting her away from the house for a couple hours was healthy. Then suddenly she seemed to stop paying attention and stopped asking questions. She used to ask, 'what is the name of this street we are on?' This stopped. Now she doesn't realize what's happening. Restaurants are no more. I don't want to deal with the mess or the look.

Ma, complaining about how I did something which was only done the way it was for her safety. To hear "don't do that" from Ma ....who needs this?

The remarks from Ma about how I'm handling her are tough to take. Like I'm trying to hurt her. I do all I can to move her in a way that is the safest for me and her.

In the throes of Alzheimer's disease, Ma would occasionally think that I was trying to cause her harm. There were many days when I could hear talk like this and shrug it off with some attempted humor. But then there were days I had no tolerance for such an assertion, and I would hurry to finish my job so I could get away.

People don't know how hard this is. No one knows unless you are doing it. Do it themselves if they feel like they can do better. I don't need criticism. People come and go here but they are not here for it all. They just get a sample in their short stay here. Let them do it all from morning till night for a week or two or three...the diaper changes, the butt wiping, moving Ma around. See what they think then.

I would feel resentment toward those who could live a normal life by coming and going as they pleased without being restrained by some heavy responsibility. I felt tied to the house, with no privacy and little opportunity to do anything I wanted to do.

Acquaintances would come for a few hours and while they were nice to Ma, they would offer suggestions that had long ago been attempted. I had no patience to hear it and took it as criticism. I was very defensive.

The cordialness is gone. This is like taking care of a baby or a pet. The odors, the smells, being peed on, dealing with poop.

This was my mother. How could I refer to her as a pet? Nurturing the mother-son relationship more would have helped in this regard. I needed to be reminded of what I was doing and who I was doing it for. My calibration, my compass was lost. I was not in the right frame of mind.

I want to remember what her hands look and feel like. How she puts her hand to her face. How she looks. She is beautiful, but so tired.

How long are her days? The boredom must be relentless. I come and I go. She is here all day confined to 100 square feet of space. How does she do it?

Ma's mind wanders, finding the correct path less and less frequently. But when she does it's a wonderful thing. The window of opportunity to hold a normal conversation with her is closing. I better say what I want to say before it is too late.

Her arm and leg do not cooperate. I hate them. They get in the way. They make things harder. Why do I have to deal with this?

The contrast in emotion I was feeling from day to day was astounding. When I would wake up the next morning and see what I had written about my feelings the night before, they almost seemed out of character for me. Fatigue and stress were reduced by a good night's sleep, but the process would repeat again the next day.

What is going on in her head? Does she still hear me? She seems to at times. She asked if I was going to marry Darlene. Wow where did that come from? There are things happening in there. She does know what's going on.

This was a brief mother–son moment, the type of thing that had been missing for so long. This occurred in the bathroom where we would be closer than any other time during the day. Ma was alert for a brief period. I believe Ma knew she was leaving soon.

Her right hand twitches and shakes like never before. The veins are more apparent. She is losing some weight. She does not eat well. We try to give as much fluid as she can take.

I look into her room in the morning when she is sleeping and I wish at times it was different. She is still breathing. Another day of this. How long can I go on with this? What am I missing?

Watching her struggle over the years has been heartbreaking. Living alone all those years and the falls. The heat and the cold in her house. The loneliness and boredom. How did she do it? It makes me feel closer to her. I was so glad to be able to take her away from that 10 years ago. But that was her home. Her memories were there. I took her away from what was important to her.

I use this caregiving thing to my benefit at times. To get out of social things I don't want to do, or to excuse myself from some obligation. Selfishness maybe but I don't care.

Ma is tired. She slumps. I prop her up and she slumps again.

Feel safe Ma. Feel secure. Don't be afraid. It's all okay.

Even the person closest to me doesn't get it. She doesn't anticipate my need to be home. It's a strain to have to be home at a certain time and worse when I have to remind everyone of this.

It was hard to have a relationship and care for Ma at the same time. Darlene helped me tremendously over the years. I didn't express this to her at the time and I should have. Without her this would have been harder. Ma enjoyed her and often perked up when she was around. I'm indebted.

Closing doors, taking the knobs off the stove. Don't have to do that now. I just put Ma in the recliner and her immobility gives me freedom. Angry at having to be home early, and feeling guilty when I don't get there, but it fades quickly when I open the door and see Ma sleeping in the recliner. Does she know? Does she put up with this without complaining so I can "have a life?"

I'm angry that people don't know. Others are watching TV, getting ready for bed. I'm in the bathroom with Ma. I want to be here but I don't want to be here. I wish I didn't have to be her caregiver and that I could be more of a son. The two don't mix.

The last thing I remember my dad saying was, 'who is going to take care of Ma?' Would he be happy and proud of how long Ma has survived? 25 years now since his death. It would be nice if he could see.

Ma is not a churchgoer. I wonder if I should have found a place for her to go to on Sundays. There were always things to do though...my things. I regret this some. I think it could have given her some comfort because she knows she is fading.

The array of emotion about all of this...from being sick and tired of doing this to not wanting it to stop...not wanting her to be gone.

The lost relationship is what I miss the most. Looking forward to seeing her. Engaging conversation, seeing her smile and twist the corner of the page with her fingers like she used to do. I miss that. Now I'm changing her clothes in silence, going through the motions, to be done with it. Maybe I'll ask what shirt she'd like to wear. I should do that more. Out of bed into the wheelchair, out to the kitchen for meds, breakfast and into the living room for TV. No talk, no conversation. I've lost it. This is wrong.

I feel I'm going through a grieving process while Ma is alive. Grieving the loss of our relationship, the loss of normal mental health, the loss of her spirit. This grief doesn't feel like a bad thing. It feels normal.

I was privileged to be in the position where I could see her every day. Even to do small things for her like get her ice cream or a drink felt good. The verbal responses from Ma were shorter and less frequent, but still rewarding. When she was more alert and I was in the proper mood, I would attempt to engage her in a conversation. They were short but very nice.

"My meds," Ma said this morning. Again always reminds me about her medication. I've been doing this for 9 years. I don't need a reminder. Stop.

I didn't react well to the comment Ma made. Instead of being annoyed, I should have been thankful she was communicating and given her praise.

'Baths take an hour. I don't look forward to them, only the finish. I like to wash Ma's hair because she seems to enjoy that part of it…the scrubbing of her scalp. The rest of the routine is a debate about the

temperature of the water and whether she would fall off the stool in the shower.'

At times, I find myself to be slower, like the pace of the world has slowed. When I feel this way I'm more patient with Ma. Not having so much to do on a particular day makes a difference. I like these days. I can sit with her and wait patiently as she tries to eat. I believe I am in the grieving process. It feels natural. Part of getting ready. I talk to Ma more on these days. Please don't let this wear off.

The ice cream at the end of the day seems to perk Ma up. After a day of sleeping and little eating or talking it was good to see Ma enjoying something.

Not recognizing family so much anymore. Forgetting names maybe more like it. She surely wants to say the name but it doesn't come to her easy.

I didn't know what was happening in her mind. She was locked in silence much of the time. Her eyes may have appeared blank but there was likely a lot happening behind them. This was confirmed for me later 3 or 4 days before her death.

Open your mouth Ma so I can feed you! What makes your jaw lock down like that? Waiting forever just to get the straw in her mouth and then waiting more to see the juice go up the straw into her mouth…God it's like torture at times. My arm gets tired. Shouldn't be this way. Shouldn't be this hard.

Waiting for that fluid to go up the straw into Ma's mouth meant to me that she was getting something into her system, and that she wanted to continue. It was anticipated and a relief to see. The lag time between the straw going into her mouth and seeing the fluid rise up the straw became greater and greater. This would try my patience. I would give up and come back in a few minutes.

Ma is so tired. How long can a body go on like this? Quality of life? I feel helpless. I'd like to take her out but she even refuses to go outside. I'll take her anyway.

What does she know, feel, hear?

She doesn't/won't talk. "Ma, do you want toast?" No answer, just a stare. Only stares this morning. Then suddenly while pushing her to the living room, "Oh John." What does that mean? Does she think I'm trying to hurt her?

Every night as I tuck Ma in, I tell her what day tomorrow would be. "Tomorrow is Monday Ma," I say tonight. "Tomorrow is Monday," Ma responds. Yahoo…there is something still there.

Sleeves don't slide on or off. Foot gets caught in PJ bottoms. She resists. On the way to trash can with diaper, "I've had it."

That walk to the trash can with Ma's diaper was only about fifty feet, but time enough for so many of those disturbing thoughts to occur.

"Goodnight Ma," "Goodnight John," -- The last four words spoken between us each day for the last 9-and-one-half years. I used to give Ma a little kiss on the forehead before bed each night. That was up until 4 or 5 years ago. Don't know why I don't do that anymore. Almost afraid to start again.

I was afraid of Ma finally passing away. I kept my distance possibly to protect my emotions. I knew it was going to hurt. I have always been protective of Ma, from the time I was a kid. Her passing was not something I could face easily, yet still I wanted the work to be done. The contradicting emotions were surprisingly strong in each direction.

Ma having trouble speaking. Then suddenly she says "The towel." I don't know what that means.

Ma not willing to open her mouth for oatmeal, but does so for her straw. She always used to complain that her oatmeal was too hot when it wasn't. This was just her way of protecting herself. This means she is using a thought process. That's good.' But I know the oatmeal is not too hot. I touch it to her lips. She still does not open. That's bad. Come on, I need to get going.

Difficulty eating. Won't open mouth. Sleeping most of day. I have no patience. My friend comes along and makes her something different to eat. Ma eats. She is sweet and nice to her. Makes me feel both mad and ineffective. Mad because she acts like it's so easy. Ineffective because I couldn't get her to eat.

There were times when my relationship with Darlene would affect my care of Ma. Giving attention to two people was a strain. Bills, work, life certainly had an effect also, but it seemed that relationship trouble had the most effect on what I had to do with Ma. If I was short, or less patient than usual, because of something having to do with Darlene, I would feel guilty about this afterward. I'd say to myself, "I'm never going to let that happen again." But I did.

She talks so little now. I want to remember what she says. Ma on the toilet. "Did you poop Ma?" "I don't remember", she says.

91

Bony facial anatomy becoming more prominent. Again, sleeping much of the day. She reaches toward the sky with her right hand. What is she seeing?

Why do I write here? Because I feel I need to. As a tribute to her. And as a lesson. Don't lose sight of who this is....my mom.

Another trip to the edge. Another TIA. Tone changes. Left arm and leg relaxed. Sleeping much of the time. Eyes change color. This renews my patience, my desire to care. Scary. Makes me sad. Don't want to lose her. Want her comfortable.

Family here. She doesn't know who they are without cues. We have a new rule. Ma is not required to remember names anymore. The pressure is off. Family presence matters. It all matters.

She ate well tonight. Peaches. "Where did you get those?" she asks. Back from oblivion. How long will this last this time? It's been several months since incident in March when the fixed stare occurred. Unresponsive. Rapid shallow breaths.

She wouldn't eat her ice cream tonight. Wouldn't open her mouth. Maintain, John. Then after putting her to bed, after dealing with poop and being gentle, she asks, "Why do you do this?"

Where once there were off-the-wall questions or comments from Ma, there is now very little talk. She used to say "There is a cat over there," or "What's in that box?" when there was no box or cat. These used to bother me because I'd have to explain them away. Now there is a blank stare, with occasional fleeting eye movement, gazing at the wall or floor, the TV on but no attention to it. I wish there were those questions again because silence is all there is now. No verbal communication. The little arm movements to help me put her shirt on, the little movements she would make to make my job easier, they are gone. I talk to her now without expecting a reply. This makes it easier.

Previously Ma and I had an understood routine with dressing and undressing. No words were needed. Ma knew what to do to help. She knew where to put her right hand to help with the left at the perfect time to make my job easier. She knew exactly when to grasp my arm and when to release. Ma knew that when I put my hands under her arms it was time to push off with her right leg for standing. I would hold her up in a standing position from her side with my left arm while I did what I had to do for cleaning and dressing her with my right. She did what she could do to help.

"It's a hot day outside Ma," I said to her today. I don't know what gets into her brain. I hope something. "Your nails need clipping." No comeback comments. No glancing at her nails. No reaction, but it's okay. She looks so frail.

I don't know what's going on in there, or if she is trying to get out. I can only behave and communicate as if there is something there. When Ma speaks, it is only in partial sentences. She struggles to finish. She wants to finish but can't. Hurts to see this. Her arms cross more in an unusual way.

"What are you..." Ma says.

"Why are you..."

What is she trying to say?

"I am..." Again, stopping.

She can't tell me if she likes or doesn't like something, whether she is comfortable or not. Then I ask her if she likes something and she reacts with a nod. How nice to get a reaction.

"Where is that little girl?" she asks.

"Don't know what you mean Ma."

"About 12 years old," she states.

So many thoughts stuck in her head. They only get halfway out. I say goodnight to her as I do always, and exit her room. I'm waiting for the response that has come all these years but is now stuck in her head. I know she must want to respond, but it doesn't come. How awful to want to say something but can't and then have the person you want to say it to leave before it can be said. I don't have the patience to wait but I do listen. Oh well that's the way it goes. I'm gone.

I would notice Ma's right arm crossing her body in an odd manner more frequently. Her left arm was contracted against her stomach, but I'd find her right arm positioned across the left so much so that I'd have to pull it back across to the right side. I don't know if she was in pain. She didn't seem to be. I learned later that this could have been a form of *decerebration rigidity*, a reflex or involuntary movement seen in some people near death.

Does she know she is declining? Does she feel it? Does she detect my frustration, like when I'm feeding her and she doesn't open her mouth? She wants to but just can't make the muscles work. She can tell I'm frustrated but neither of us can say we are sorry. How sad.

Just a little more Ma. Come on, you can do it. Five more bites. Half a cup more of juice.

A lot of effort was put into getting Ma to eat. When I was smart about it, I'd just walk away and come back in a few minutes, and things seemed to be easier. Darlene was very helpful attempting to feed Ma. I didn't express enough appreciation for her help at the time.

Darlene would buy Ma treats that she knew Ma enjoyed. She was very soft and kind to Ma, giving her a kiss at night and telling Ma she loved her. Ma and I did not have that relationship. Oddly enough, I was afraid that I would cry if I tried to kiss Ma on the forehead.

She deserves to be comfortable and cared for properly. 10 years ago, I made the decision to take over her life. I thought it was best. I did not want to see anymore struggle or injury. Is she struggling now, again? Boredom, slow physical decline, starvation. Are these the terms she would have accepted if she were in her right mind?

"Do you want some ice cream Ma?" "Sure," she responds. Some calm water for Ma. Opening her mouth to eat. Responsive. Eyes open. What does this mean?

I find myself to be attentive at times but disconnected at others. I look for distractions, anything so I don't have to deal with what is in front of me.

My cell phone kept me from being as attentive to my mom as I could have been. It was a distraction, entertainment for me. This kept me from interacting with Ma and promptly attending to her needs. I wish I could have back every moment of delay caused by me and my cell phone.

Getting her up this morning, Saturday. "The gardeners are here Ma." "The gardeners!" she perks up. Wow, what a response. I'm putting her shirt on and she says, "Wait," I say "Wait for what Ma?" I said rather curtly. "Wait for me to catch up," Ma replies.

Where was my sensitivity and tenderness toward Ma? What possessed me to act that way toward her?

The gardeners' blower is going. I ask Ma if she can hear the gardeners. Ma says, "Who cannot hear the gardeners?" One of the few things that separate one day from another for Ma has been the gardener on Saturday, but she has been unresponsive to this for weeks.

A short while later, Ma says "I want to go home." Oh, my god, after all this time she still holds onto that hope. "To Pittsburg?" I say, her hometown in Northern California. "Yes", she says. Where is this coming from? Is this the end?

After a good day, a bad. Minimal response. No hand movements. Slumped, bottom lip protruding. Difficulty taking fluids. Sleep all day. I found myself annoyed by this, angry. Why this? Have to work to get food into her mouth again.

Three-day trip to Cambria. Me and Darlene. Ma at home with caregiver. Expensive but worthwhile. Felt like I needed it. Wasn't really worried about Ma. Should I feel guilty? Ma up in chair when I got home at 9 pm. Initially, I was hoping she would be in bed...one more night's reprieve...but I wasn't too disappointed. Gave me a chance to interact some and give her some ice cream. All in all, a good trip. Feel de-stressed some. What will tomorrow bring?

Ma very quiet today. Eyes seem a bit more gray than blue. Blank stares. Delayed responses and not eating much. Appears not just tired but disconnected.

I wonder what it must feel like inside to know you are going down, that there will be no recovery as there has been in the past. Like sliding off a table with no grip available.

No talk today. I ask questions, not really expecting a reply. Maybe she knows what to say but the connection to the mouth does not work.

Alone, Ma sits in her recliner. The TV is on but who knows what Ma sees or hears? I feel the need to provide entertainment but I don't know what to do. I feel pressure from others to do social things and be away from home. Duffy boat ride. Too long to be away, but I go. I think about Ma while out there. When I get home, there is no talk. Ma has been alone for 4 hours. Too long. I give her all the water I can. She is thirsty and sips through the straw, but not like she used to. I've become attuned to the speed at which the fluid goes up the straw. I feel I need to stay with her more.

Small movements are traumatic for Ma. I turn her wheelchair, and Ma responds "Oh John," in a fearful manner. Pushing the wheelchair …she must feel I'm going 100 mph. Fear. She ate well today. Tuna, and of course ice cream. No talk. She wants to but can't get the words out.

I have flashbacks of trips with Ma and the kids while she has been with me. Las Vegas. The kids' games. The rides home from the kids' house with Ma. Lots of them. We used to do so much more than we do now.

Next weekend…10 years with Ma.

After not talking most of the day, Ma said, "I just ran next to…." "Are you alright Ma?" I ask. "I'm alright," Ma responds. I want to believe her.

The boredom, the routine. Up out of bed, dressed, breakfast, recliner, lunch, dinner, undressed, bed. How can a person not die from the boredom?

"Any pains tonight Ma?" 3 or 4 minutes pass. I tap on her knee to break her out of her stare. "Ma, do you have any pain?" Finally, "Is there water on the floor?" It is easy for me to answer. I feel no aggravation. I hold her hand some. She doesn't exactly respond to my grasp, but she does not pull away either.

Four or five more days until 10 years with Ma.

Heard from caregiver that Ma ate poorly and slept most of the day. When I got home she was resting comfortably with her eyes open, looking pretty good. She did not respond to my questions though. I asked later if she wanted ice cream, and she labored out a soft yes. Fed her the ice cream and off to the bathroom. I asked her if she hurt. No response. I asked if her tummy hurt. She softly said "no." Does your bladder hurt? "No." Does your head hurt? "No." "Well that's good, Ma. You don't hurt." Yes, that seems to be," she says. I tell her that this weekend will be 10 years with me here. She says, "That's a long time." She is awake. Let's keep going. I ask, "Do you still consider yourself to be a Northern California girl?" "Yes, I prefer Northern California." WOW! A conversation. So nice when she comes out of the fog.

Ma often slept during the day for prolonged periods which certainly must have affected her sleep at night. I would go into her room at night sometimes and find her awake staring at the ceiling or trying to reach up for something. I tried to reassure her that everything was fine, she didn't have to worry.

Ma did not display signs of Sundowner Syndrome, seen commonly in those with dementia. Ma did not become irritable or angry in the evening hours. On many occasions, she was more alert and talkative during the evening hours, but never verbally aggressive.

I have thought on occasion that I should have taken Ma back to her house, where her memories are, so she could live out her days there. I think that would have been nice.

Sunday, 9/6/15. Ma's 10-year anniversary of being with me. I was so naive 10 years ago thinking I was doing a good thing. I wonder now. Is she suffering? Living the most days possible...is this the best thing?

Ma will say, 'I think you....'. Her mind gets stuck and she can't finish. I believe she thinks I'm trying to abuse her at times. I take her to the kid's house for dinner. She doesn't do much but sleep there. Does she hear me complain about how hard it is to get her in the car? What a fool I am for saying this aloud. I don't want her to think she is a burden on me. I wanted to do this.

This is so frustrating. And draining. The relationship between Ma and I...the fun little conversations, the kidding, the happy to be in the same room feelings...they are gone. Now she is a person sitting in a wheelchair who I feed and water. She may or may not know what it takes to care for her. That's not so important. I hope, but doubt, she knows that I'm doing this out of love for her. If she doesn't know this, then fine. I'm still obligated to take good care of her.

Another day, out of bed, dressed, to the kitchen, cranberry juice and a hair comb, medications, oatmeal and maybe a piece of toast. All in all, not bad. What would my father think?

Eating well, opening mouth today. What a difference that makes. Last night would not open mouth. "You are being difficult," I told her. "You're difficult," she responded. Ah, a response.

This morning, no verbal responses until... "Do you want toast Ma?"

"Yes."

"Can you do that by yourself?" I ask if she can eat her toast without help.

"Well I don't know."

"Okay."

She did it. "Good job Ma. You are doing good today."

She is scared when I move her. Any movement pushing her in the wheelchair, transferring her to the toilet...it is all scary. She has no control.

There is more there than we think. She senses, she thinks, she feels. It may be clouded in fog at times but she is there. She can't express like she'd like, respond like she'd like, but she is there.

Would not open mouth...no response...eyes open....would not suck through straw. Leave her be. Don't express anger or frustration. Give it a minute or two and come back.

She sucks up the straw.

"Good, Ma."

She gets stuck. I have to realize this. Go with the flow.

I do not want anyone to care for me like this.

As long as Ma sucks fluid up the straw into her mouth....is this the clue that she wants to continue on? When this one little thing stops, is that the sign.

Having her grasp the bed when I'm trying to move her in bed, such a chore sometimes. She is fearful. I have to say, "Relax Ma, this is not that hard". But of course, it is for her.

Fluid became Ma's primary source of nourishment. I became fixated on waiting for fluid to go up the straw. Ensure and cranberry juice were the norms. Her sucking and swallowing functions were an important sign to me that things were still working and she wanted to go on.

Ma very quiet. No talking. Then suddenly she will say something- usually yes or no in response to a question. She will not open her mouth on command. She must want to, just can't. It's in there, rattling around in her head, looking for an opening to come out. Darlene feeding Ma. She talks to Ma. Ma responds. I wonder if she just got lucky or is it me? I wonder how Ma sees me. Does she know who I am or am I just a stranger to her now?

Ma with a few good nights being talkative, alert. Better than during the day. Then two to three days bad. Pushing fluids. She will not eat well. Ma asked if a priest came to the house. When I put her to bed I asked, "So you saw a priest here Ma?" She said, "Well why couldn't there be?"

I told the hospice person about the priest comment and she said she would ask Ma if she wanted a priest to come see her.

The hospice clergy person was very comforting. I felt some relief, with her presence there, for not having taken Ma to church more. We were not a religious family but Ma had indicated some interest over the last few years.

My ex-wife Nikki asked Ma if she wanted to pray with her. Ma responded yes.

Ma's birthday weekend... 86 years old. Family here on Saturday...brother and sister with their spouses. Ma had a good Friday night, but very sleepy Saturday and Sunday. Does she know they are here? Family sees the decline. What does Ma think when they come over to hold her hand? Is there happiness or sadness? I want to tell Ma she should feel proud. I hope she feels that. Little reaction. Blank stares. Sleeping. Sad to know this may be the last time they see her alive. No response with birthday cake. Does it make her sad when they leave and say goodbye? Can't tell. Hope not.

Ma 86 years old. She was sixty when my dad died and asked, "Who is going to care for Ma?" I hope he can see that she has done well. 15 years on her own she lived. Such a survivor. So tough. She did very well. I want her to know this. Pick a time to let her know. Don't wait. She should be so proud.'

I caught Ma awake. I was able to tell her how proud she should be of her kids. How she lived 15 years on her own. She was attentive. This was nice. Her eyes were open. She asked about Charlie.

Charlie was an uncle of hers who had died many years earlier.

Recertification nurse came to visit Ma to renew Hospice order. She left me a message and told me to call her. She said a few things. First, that Ma was being cared for very well. That she was lucky to have me. That made my throat tighten. I said we just didn't want her to be in a nursing home.

When Ma's eyes are open, we try to talk. "Are you good Ma?"

"I'm good," she will respond on a good day. I told her again she should be proud of living alone those 15 years after dad died. She said she was.

I hold her hand. She gives back a good grasp, before she lets go and reaches up into the air for something only she can see. Oh, Ma. Eggnog for dessert tonight. Ma drank it up good.

Very little talking today. It's Saturday again. Gardeners here but no response from Ma. The family has come and gone. I get it that people don't get it. You can't relate to something you don't do. Back to the routine, the boredom.

Ma is precious. She should be happy. It's ok that this is hard. I will miss it when it is gone. Ma in bed in the next room. She is warm and safe. What will it be like when she is not here anymore?

Very little talk but that's Ok. I talk as if she hears everything.

No response used to frustrate me. No need to be frustrated. If she could talk more, I'm sure she would. All is fine. She is here, at home, being cared for. She is not alone or in a strange place, hearing strange noises. Sleep good Ma.

Quiet day, occasionally responsive. Ma seemed to respond to Breanna (my daughter). Buttons. Remember how much they use to bother me.

Very few sentences from Ma. One/two-word answers. Occasionally she will repeat part of a phrase or comment someone will say. That has to be frustrating for her. I don't want her to feel that way.

"I need to change my clothes," Ma said before bed tonight. She never said anything like this before. Diaper dirty. It's a struggle to change her diaper and she gets scared. I hope she wasn't afraid to say

that. She has never been demanding in any way. Probably hard for her to say this.

Does she feel she is a burden? I hope not. Does she feel ashamed? I hope not. She doesn't deserve to, yet I didn't take a moment so say "No problem Ma," when it came to that diaper. I should have said something.

I tell her to sleep good, and that tomorrow is Saturday. No response. Her eyes were open but closed immediately. Tell her you love her. Tell her before it's too late.

Red bottom. Is her skin breaking down? She does not open her mouth well. I have to force the straw into her mouth. Sucking up the straw becoming more difficult.

Ma's skin was very healthy for the most part, especially considering how much time she spent sitting. Ma was very in tune to the health of her skin. She knew that sores were a bad sign and whenever we suspected one may be starting she took great interest in asking how it was doing.

Saturday, October 31st. No words from Ma today. Seemingly more contracted. Her arms were crossed. Knees tightly together. Curled up in her chair. No verbal responses. Once in her chair she drank well, ate poorly. Another day toward the end.

Is Ma hungry? How must that feel to think your mouth is open but it isn't. Then to have me say over and over, "open your mouth, Ma."

Ma was changing physically with her decreased intake of food. She had lost weight and her skin was loose. Bony prominences were more apparent. The crossing of her arm and stiffness of her legs was more frequent. She was talking less and less and sleeping more. Hospice was coming 2 to 3 days a week for bathing and nursing visits. Ma's heart rate and blood pressure were good. She had no pain. Ma's regular caregiver, Paula, was communicating with me every day about any changes in Ma.

Good day for Ma. Awake, talked, ate and drank well. She had a bath done today by hospice.

"Did you have a bath today Ma?"

"The last time I had a bath was with George."

"Who is George?"

"One of the farm hands."

"Where are you Ma?"

"The three musketeers."

"Every time I move my arm... She never finishes.

"Goodnight Ma. Sleep good."

"Goodnight John"

I don't get frustrated when Ma fails to reciprocate with a conversation. When she does, it's just an extra nice thing.'

Tonight, when I put Ma to bed and tucked her in, I told her that I came into the room early this morning before I left and found her with face buried face down, nose into the pillow. Must have been hard to breathe. I told her I moved the pillow and readjusted her. No response. I said goodnight, sleep good, and left the room. Before I got too far I heard Ma say "Thanks for the nose job." I laughed.

***

This next journal entry was my last before Ma's death. It describes our last night in the bathroom.

Sunday night November 8th, as I was attempting to lift Ma out of her chair to transfer to the toilet, she grabbed the wheelchair. I could feel the extra weight as I was trying to lift her. She was lifting the wheelchair off the floor as I stood her up. I could not sit her back down because the chair was tilted. Her feet then began to slip from underneath her.

I tried to block them with my left leg as I tried to knock the wheelchair out of Ma's hand. We were slowly heading toward the floor. I still had to pull her diaper down which somehow I did. Ma must have been very scared. I did not want her to go to the floor because there was some bowel movement that had landed on the floor. I finally dislodged the wheelchair from her hand and placed her up onto the toilet.

I walked out to the garage and paced a bit. My heart was beating fast and I was breathing heavily. That was physically stressful for both me and Ma, but I also felt anger. I waited a few minutes, again wondering how much more of this I can do.

I went back into the bathroom and I outstretched my arms and asked, "What was that?" Ma just turned her head right and then left and then right, looking up at me. I'll never forget it. What was wrong with me? How could I say that to her?

Ma had loose bowel movement that had gone down her legs. It took a while to clean. Once done, I transferred her back to the wheelchair, and during this transfer I noticed she had no power in her right leg. She

106

would always try to help with her right leg. Virtually no standing ability. What a night.

What I didn't say in this journal entry was just as important as what was said. I gave great detail, as it was fresh in my head, but I couldn't admit my true feelings that I had done something wrong. Ma's left leg was limp as I transferred her back to bed. She could hardly stand up on her right. That was not normally the case. The complete lack of standing ability was unusual. I should have been more alarmed about this than I was. I was afraid to fully recognize what had just happened.

The next day, Paula the caregiver texted me at about 10 A.M.:

John, I believe Charlotte may have had a stroke over the weekend. She woke up with severe diarrhea. I couldn't get her to eat or drink anything. She kept retching, like she wanted to throw up but didn't. It was unusually difficult to dress her. She has no control over her legs and her speech is very garbled and not sure if she has a stuffy nose. Maybe she is coming down with the flu but I can always understand her speech, but not today. I moved her to the recliner and she went right to sleep. Will wake her in a bit to see if I can get her to drink and eat something.

I got home from work around one. As soon as I walked in and saw Ma I knew this was going to be the end. She was sitting slumped but upright, not leaning to the left as she normally would. She never sits upright unless there is something wrong or she is injured. Her breathing was rapid and shallow.

The caregiver gave me an update as I knelt in front of Ma. I don't know for sure if she knew I was there. I grabbed her hand and it felt weak, limp, and clammy. Her eyes were open but gray in color.

I opened her right nostril which seemed to be stuck closed. This seemed to ease up her breathing some. She turned her head slightly and looked at me when I did this, as if to say thank you. She could not speak.

Everything was different. I thought, "Oh Ma, I'm so sorry." The night before in the bathroom was too much. All the nights over the past ten years, rolling Ma into the bathroom and transferring her to the toilet, it was a routine. Never was there a night like the last night.

I felt severe guilt that I should have handled the situation differently. I should have done better. The fear and the stress Ma must have felt, dangling in the air, not knowing what was happening. She was fine before we went into the bathroom. I had given her some leftover stuffing with cranberry just before bed and she ate it fairly well.

Ma needed me that night. She needed my decision making for her well-being, but I wasn't ready. I was too impatient to deal with what was happening. I should have sat Ma back down in the chair as soon as I noticed she was gripping the chair. I didn't have the patience to do something twice, so I forged ahead and compromised Ma's safety. I just wanted to be done.

Unfortunately, Ma probably broke her left hip sometime during the struggle to get Ma on the toilet. The caregiver noted a bruise on the back of her left hip, and there seemed to be a pain response from Ma when moving her left leg. That lack of tone that I noticed in her left leg when I put her to bed should have been my clue.

The hospice nurse came by to see Ma that afternoon. He said Ma most likely had another stroke. It wasn't ever said specifically, but everyone just assumed that this was Ma's final turn toward death. There was never any talk of taking her to the hospital. The ordinary procedure was palliative care, not hospitalization. I questioned this later. Ma was a fighter. Why didn't we give her more of a chance? I guess I knew the end was coming deep down, but I was refusing to totally accept it.

Oxygen was ordered and it was encouraged not to give Ma food for fear of aspiration. Ma was not responsive except for occasional eye movements. She did not respond to questions or a request to squeeze the hand. Her body was limp. But this was still only the first day after the incident.

I was disappointed in myself and felt pulled down by second thoughts over the night before in the bathroom. It was my fault that she was in her final days of life after all those years of trying to keep her safe. I haven't completely come to terms with this yet and maybe I never will.

Now I was preparing for the end. Family was notified. New instructions were given to the caregiver. I decided to move Ma's hospital bed to the living room. I knew she would be bedridden and I didn't want her to be hidden back in her room. There were going to be people around and I wanted it to be easy for all of us to see Ma. Ma was very self-conscious and she probably would have disagreed with this, but I felt it had to be done for what was approaching.

Ma would never eat again and she was given only minimal fluid. Despite hospice instructions not to, she was given scant amounts of fluid because she appeared parched and it was simply too painful to witness. She would never sit up again. Morphine was used to slow her breathing when it became too rapid. She slowly withered away. That's the only way to describe it. No food or water and her organs would begin to shut down, as the hospice nurse described.

Later, when people asked me how she passed, I would think first that I made a mistake and secondly she starved. But I didn't say that. Denying nutrition until the organs shut down seems like starvation to me. There must be a better way.

109

After four days of no nutrition, a hospice nurse came to give Ma a brief bath. I was present as were a few family members. We strategized together how we would turn Ma to not cause pain in her left hip. She was basically unresponsive up to this point except when it came to pain. Slight movement of her left leg would produce a slight facial grimace. We wanted to be very careful.

As we started to turn Ma, we noticed some skin break down on the bony prominences of her back. We talked about these spots aloud. When mention of a "sore" was made, Ma opened her eyes and looked right at me. I was taken aback by this. There was a look of concern. It was not a look of pain; I was familiar with her expression of pain. It was a troubled, distressed look. Ma heard the talk of sores. She was always afraid of her skin breaking down. She knew that was not a good thing and she reacted.

Ma was aware of what was happening around her even though there were no outward signs that was the case. She could hear what we were saying. This was 3 days prior to her death, in the so-called active phase of dying. Touch can be felt and spoken word can be heard. There can be mental processing, feeling and emotion present up to the very end.

I will never forget this look on Ma's face. I tried to reassure her that everything was okay, but the word was already out. I wished that nothing had been said and that we had left her alone that day.

Ma was home. She was not alone in some ward of a hospital or nursing home. She was around family who brushed her hair, held her hand and spoke into her ear. We repositioned her for comfort and skin protection. She was loved. As the hospice nurse would say later, "This is the way to go." We felt she could sense our presence even though we did not expect a response from her.

We played music for Ma. The "oldies" were what she liked. There was one song by Doris Day that seemed perfect for Ma. It was the song *Que Sera Sera*. I know Ma could hear these songs. She loved listening to such music.

My two daughters were at Ma's bedside one afternoon three days prior to her death. They touched her hands and caressed her hair. Ma's eyes opened just for a second. They asked her if she had pain. Ma softly said no. They asked if she was comfortable. She mouthed the response yes. This would be her very last word spoken.

We reassured Ma that everything was okay and she had nothing to worry about. Still, we felt short of words for the situation. We did some internet research on the end of life. It was suggested that the dying person be comforted with phrases like: "It's time to go home." We would tell Ma it was time to go home to be with Dad and her mama. This was just as comforting to us as I hope it was for her.

Ma seemed to respond to fluid placed in her mouth up until her last two days. We used cotton swabs soaked with water. She even seemed to actively suck on the eyedropper full of morphine. Then toward the end, there was no sucking. The morphine would just sit inside her cheek without any swallow response. Her breathing was shallow and rapid; her heartbeat was faint.

"Enough of this," I said to myself, as painful as it was. Please go, Ma. There are no worries. Be free.

***

Ma passed away on Tuesday November 17, 2015 at 9:54 pm, nine days after the incident in the bathroom.

Her last moments were remarkable. She had not opened her eyes, but for brief moments during those last few days. I was sitting at her side, holding her hand. The family was there watching TV, waiting.

I opened one of Ma's eyes with my finger, maybe just to see if she would respond. Her eye was blue, not gray. I didn't want to disturb her, so I let it close. A moment later Ma opened both eyes very wide. I remarked to everyone, "Look, Ma's eyes are open."

Everyone rushed over to her bedside. She was awake like she had not been for the nine previous days. I supported her head. After a moment of maybe five seconds, just enough time for all of us to say we loved her, she took her last breath. As the color drained from her lip, it turned from pink to gray. Her eyes closed. Her chest became silent. She was gone.

We were all shocked, amazed by what just happened. This rapidly turned into a great sense of relief for Ma. Her struggle was over. We hugged each other and gave Ma a touch or a kiss each in our own way.

We had put a batch of balloons together with messages from all of us tucked inside. We went out front and released the balloons into the night with only a few words said but lots of tears and hugs. We were all so happy for Ma. Her spirit was now free.

**

Over the next few days, weeks and months, I replayed the incident in the bathroom over and over and felt that she would still be alive if I'd handled it better. My family told me that I shouldn't feel bad about that night, that it was an accident. But I know it could have been different if I had not been so exhausted with the caregiving process.

To this day I don't have a great sense of relief over not having to physically perform the tasks needed to care for Ma. I miss the routines. I miss seeing her in that recliner and having her present there in my home. Sure, I can come and go as I please now, but if I feel any relief at all, it's in the fact that Ma is now at rest.

I touch Ma's pictures and think about my brother and sister and me. Ma deserves so much love and respect for a job well done. I tell Ma so and I tell her I'm sorry.

Was it the right thing to do, bringing Ma in with me? Yes. She benefited from being with family and we benefited from having her in our lives. We had many good times together. She was warm, fed, cleaned, and looked after. I just wish my "job" hadn't interfered with the relationship we had as mother and son.

Caring for Ma all those years allows me to feel this great sense of loss. I gladly accept it. Because of our time together, Ma lives inside of me in a way no one will ever know or understand.

CAREGIVING AND THE CAREGIVER

Caring for a family member becomes necessary for many reasons. Cancer, stroke, heart disease, pulmonary (lung) disease, organ failure, diabetes, broken bones or arthritis, mental illness or Alzheimer's disease. The experience with my mom included stroke and Alzheimer's disease.

Becoming a caregiver for a loved one can be by choice or not. I chose to care for my mom. I saw her struggle and I wanted her life to be safer and easier. Many people are forced to become caregivers. The reason one becomes a care provider for a family member or loved one can determine the quality of experience for the caregiver.

Customs, oaths, and vows influence the dependence of one person on another during the time of need or illness. We are supposed to care for our 'own blood' when the situation demands it. This expectation can be a double-edged sword, sending life into a previously unknown and unexpected direction.

When you care for the parent who raised you, it completes the circle of life. This can be a very motivating thought for the caregiver. Depending on the circumstances, caregiving can also be a tremendous burden. For those who care for a spouse, the adage 'till death do us part' can make the decision the expected choice. But if a sense of duty is the main motivating factor, compassionate care may be in short supply. Caring for a child who has no independence draws on the existing bond between parent and offspring, but at a price of the parents' freedom. Whether one becomes a caregiver by choice or necessity has a significant impact on the stress level and overall satisfaction with the caregiving process.

Caregiving for reasons of love, devotion, togetherness and spiritual fulfillment tends to be a more positive experience for the caregiver. Caregiving can, and in many cases, does add meaning and quality to the life of the one providing care. About one-third of caregivers report neither strain nor negative impact upon their life from caregiving. This work makes them feel happy, productive and needed, adding to their overall health and quality of life.

When done from a sense of duty, guilt, greed or secondary gain, the outcome can be less desirable in terms of quality and compassion. Quality of care is the most important factor negatively affected by these motivations. When family economics, the need for constant supervision of the family member or the lack of anyone else to help with the job forces an already disinterested individual to make sacrifices, this can lead to an unsafe and unhealthy environment for the care recipient.

Quality of life issues for the caregiver are impacted by several specific factors. These include how many hours of caregiving are required, the level of care needed and whether the caregiver is also employed. Statistics show that those involved with caregiving greater than 21 hours a week have an increased incidence of stress-related issues. Care recipient health problems associated with dementia, cancer, and advancing age are the more difficult issues for caregivers to manage, with dementia being the most difficult of these. Employed caregivers may have to cut their hours at work, take frequent time off, or quit their jobs entirely to provide the care needed and thus incur financial hardship.

Caregivers are known to experience symptoms like those in chronically stressful situations. Physical and psychological changes may take place if the caregiver continues without needed rest or assistance. Anxiety, depression, worry, and loneliness are common psychological stressors. Social isolation and extreme feelings of resentment can compound these conditions without a method in place to express emotions. Physical manifestations that may accompany the caregiving role include fatigue, weight gain and an increased frequency of illness.

Burnout of caregivers is a well-documented condition and something that affected me in my work with Ma. I was too busy to detect the undermining effects until it was too late. The damage had been done and my compassion waned at times.

The symptoms of caregiver burnout are like those of stress and depression. They include:

* Withdrawal from friends and family

* Loss of interest in activities previously enjoyed

* Feeling blue, irritable, hopeless, and helpless

* Changes in appetite, weight, or both

* Changes in sleep patterns

* Getting sick more often

* Feelings of wanting to hurt yourself or the person you are caring for

* Emotional and physical exhaustion

* Irritability

* Excessive use of alcohol and/or sleep medications

Often the caregiver is left alone with these symptoms and feelings. They are forced to advocate for themselves to receive help but are embarrassed to do so. How and to whom can they relate such emotions?

The journal I kept helped me to express both the good and the bad, the joys and frustrations. I could vent and 'write angry' if need be without penalty. On one hand, journaling may prevent unfiltered emotions from being spoken and then regretted. On the other hand, it may be a way to present valid emotions in written form more easily than in a face to face conversation. Keeping a journal is a valuable tool that I recommend highly.

Caregivers usually will not ask for help. If they proceed down the road of burnout too far, without the help they need and deserve, the quality of care they provide will ultimately suffer. The importance of an avenue to share feelings with other family members and ask for help can't be overstated.

So much rides on the health of the caregiver. They are counted on to maintain the stability of the home, manage finances and deal with the healthcare delivery system. Add to that daily crisis management and keeping an even keel during insults or critical remarks about the quality of care provided. There may even be occasional threats of harm to the caregiver by the care recipient. The caregiver is the weakest and most important link in the chain. Other family members need to be aware of the tough row they hoe daily.

One aspect of caregiving that is vastly under-appreciated is the severely limited reward system for this work. You are, as a caregiver, directly making the life of your loved one safer and more comfortable in their hour of need, while often putting your own needs and desires aside. The nature of caregiving dictates you are usually working outside the public's view. Even your closest family members will never know all that you do. Except for visits to the doctor or social gatherings, you may remain isolated in the home, working alone. There is no one there to pat you on the back and tell you what a good job you are doing.

The work is unglamorous and downright dirty at times, with no immediate reward or favors in return. Merely the fact that you are doing something good for another human being may have to suffice as your reward. Being acknowledged by other family members for the difficult task of putting your life aside to do what you do makes the day-to-day work easier. I hope this paragraph is read and appreciated by outside family members.

The caregiver must be on the lookout for the natural changes that come with aging. Changes in mobility, sleep patterns, eating habits, orientation to space and time and the need for more frequent visits to the physician and other healthcare providers are a few examples. Loss of speech, vision, hearing, and judgment add to the demands on the caregiver by requiring closer contact with the care recipient. Loss of bowel and bladder control presents the most stress for a caregiver.

In reaction to increased physical limitation and changing life circumstances, negativity, depression, anger, and anxiety are common in the care recipient. These emotions markedly increase the level of stress on both the caregiver and care recipient and can change their relationship for the worse.

A glass-half-empty attitude in the care recipient is difficult for the caregiver to tolerate day after day. But optimism and the will to carry on are difficult for the care recipient when their health situation and ability to make decisions for themselves have been relinquished to the caregiver. It is important for the caregiver to be supportive of their loved one and try to keep their own feelings of being burdened in check.

The relationship that once existed between caregiver and care recipient will change as time together proceeds. For some, the relationship may become closer, making up for lost time. It may be a fulfilling experience for both as they coexist together. Life may be better lived together than apart.

On the other hand, doing what is right and kind for another may be unappreciated and even criticized. In this circumstance, thick skin on the part of the caregiver is a true asset. Such close contact can lead to increased, mutual animosity and tension. If the caregiver has taken on more than they can handle, the previously loving relationship can become damaged beyond repair.

I believe that caregiving for a family member, in many instances, can be harmful to the relationship between the two people involved. Hopefully, this is the exception to the rule, but the possibility does exist for this to occur. Two people living in close proximity, with differing needs, wants and deadlines, further compounded by sacrifices on the caregiver side and declining abilities on the recipient side - the ingredients are present for rising tension and stress.

To counter this tendency, I believe that the caregiver must consciously maintain a separation between their role of being the provider of care and that of being a loving family member. Only in this way can the relationship be protected from the effects of caregiving. If the closeness and tenderness of the relationship is compromised so will be the quality of care provided. This is a critically important issue that receives little, if any, attention in the literature. The quality of the relationship must be shielded from the trappings of family caregiving, and nourished as time goes on.

Photographs, "shrines," prayer, five minutes of hand holding and together mentally revisiting family history are keys to "signing out" as caregiver and "signing back in" as a loving family member. Nourishing the love and respect you have for the care recipient will pay huge dividends as time goes on.

The goal for everyone involved should be the highest quality of care possible for the family member. While the caregiver is vulnerable to the effects of caregiving, it is the care recipient who will suffer the most if proper care is not maintained. This issue is of utmost importance. Respite care for the caregiver is vital in order to assure lasting and appropriate care. It falls on outside family members to assure that the health of the caregiver is maintained so that their important work can continue with compassion and quality.

Of course, the caregiver and care recipient will have a natural bond. If, however, the caregiver becomes overly protective and hesitant to allow others into the home to observe how the family member is doing, an unhealthy situation is created. There must be honesty and transparency between the caregiver, care recipient and the outside world.

In the case of outside, paid help, regular communication and observation visits need to take place to make sure things are done correctly. Outside help is expensive but that doesn't guarantee it is providing quality care. Human nature being what it is, some people may do less and expend the least amount of effort possible when no one is looking. Unannounced visits, video cameras and regular written and verbal reports can be utilized to guarantee proper care. Defining specific responsibilities, in writing, with mutual agreement is very important.

Often, becoming a caregiver 'just happens'. It is not something planned for well in advance. If there is any preparation time for this important job, it is usually minimal. The transition between part-time to full-time caregiver may be slow and that can help with the learning process. If the responsibility arrives full force, without much warning, outside help and support are essential.

Caregiving is noble work that requires adaptation to its demands. Both the challenges and the rewards can be quite surprising. Fortunately, adaptation is a strong suit in the human race.

There is a special, unexpected result that comes with caring for a family member. Caregiving entitles you to feel things others cannot, especially when the loved one passes away. While this loss may be especially painful for you, you have a unique perspective. No one else can fully relate to what you have done, the struggles you have faced, or how you now feel. The love you exhibited in caregiving heightens the sense of loss when the caring is done. It may be hard to understand, but the depth of your sorrow means you've given in a way many cannot.

TEN YEARS OF LEARNING TOO LATE

Experience is the best teacher. My advice about caregiving comes from my ten-year experience of being the primary caregiver for my mother. Reflecting upon this experience in the months since her death has led me to some important conclusions that I feel should be shared with all family caregivers.

Caregiving will shake the foundation of who you are, prompting you to ask yourself how you arrived at the place where you think and feel the way you do. These challenges are only truly understood by those who have faced them.

How an individual reacts and adapts to caregiving will depend on their individual talents, education, beliefs and cultural background. Some are not cut out to be caregivers. Others handle it naturally and with ease. What one sees on the outside isn't necessarily what's happening on the inside of a caregiver.

In the later years, I felt as if I was traversing the underside of a cornice, defying gravity with minimal finger and foot holds. An occasional rock would fly at me from below in the form of a comment or criticism about how I was doing something. I was fearful of the next event that would pull me down, once and for all. Where was some sort of anchor or rope to secure myself?

It's said that the struggle is what counts because that is how you learn. Here is what I learned, although much of it too late. These are the things I would do differently, knowing what I know now.

1. Be prepared. Learn about caregiving.

2. Establish a routine of respite care for yourself from the beginning.

3. Do not lose sight of who you are caring for.

4. Know your limits.

5. Anticipate changes in the relationship with your loved one.

6. Understand your own emotions in the caregiving role.

7. Absorb, don't react. Flex, don't break. Guide, don't force.

8. Be careful of what, when and how you say things, but say what needs to be said.

9. Seek out community support through church, support groups, friends and neighbors.

10. Make time for fun and entertainment.

11. Let people know your honest thoughts by sharing a journal or a letter. Have family meetings.

12. Cherish yourself. You need it. You deserve it.

Be prepared. Learn about caregiving.

I highly suggest the following reading: Caregiving 101: On Being a Caregiver, by Family Caregiver Alliance, National Center on Aging, www.caregiver.org, (800 445 8106). This is an excellent summary for potential or new caregivers, and is valuable information presented in an easy to read format.

I was mad at caregiving. I wasn't mad a Ma. Frustration came from my lack of knowledge. Most families put more work into preparing for the arrival of a new puppy than I put into preparing for what was ahead of me.

Depending on the diagnosis, prognosis and functional limitations of the family member, professional help may be needed to learn patient handling techniques for transfers, ambulation and community mobility. This will make trips away from home much easier and eliminate unnecessary additional stress when going to medical appointments or other outings. Proper positioning techniques also must be learned to help prevent skin irritation and breakdown. All these skills can be taught to the caregiver by a nurse or therapist who will come to the home to provide the training. To obtain these services, you must request a home health referral from the patient's doctor.

Organization of the home for easy access to all supplies helps the caregiver avoid unnecessary steps and means they won't have to leave the side of the care recipient to fetch something that's not handy. Easy transition of the care recipient between the bed, bathroom, dining and TV areas via wheelchair, walker, or arm in arm assistance decreases the risk of falls or injury to the caregiver. It is recommended to remove throw rugs, cords, and unneeded furniture. Grab bars, non-stick surfaces, a raised commode or toilet seat, shower chair or tub transfer benches decrease the dangers in the bathroom.

Learning about dementia, specifically Alzheimer's disease, and the death and dying process eases the fear and anxiety associated with each of these. The unknown can be exceptionally frightening at the end of life. We can manage our own emotions better with added knowledge and preplanning.

Caregivers may not have the opportunity or time to research and seek appropriate medical referrals. Other family members can provide this invaluable assistance. Unfortunately, the caregiver may be hesitant to ask for help. Another family member who takes on the role to closely monitor the caregiving situation can step in to provide the needed assistance.

Establish a routine of respite care for yourself from the very beginning.

Plain and simple, this is the most important factor to consider for the long-term health of the caregiver. Please see the chapter on respite care.

Do not lose sight of whom you are caring for.

Never forget or fail to appreciate the life you shared with your family member before becoming their caregiver. Continually honoring the life that now rests in your hands will help maintain the proper perspective needed when the going gets rough. The altruistic feeling of caring for another will not hold up by itself when the demands of caregiving begin to hit home. There must be reminders available to keep you aware of why you are doing what you do.

Ma brought my brother, sister and me into the world and endured a great deal of heartache while raising us. I was always devoted to her, but my devotion lost the kindness it had at the beginning. I tried to talk myself out of being just a caregiver and into being more of a son. But fatigue often got the best of me. I needed a visual reminder, a photo or memento of our past. A quiet spot should have been set aside for me to retreat, de-stress and remember.

A 'shrine' to Ma's life and what she meant to the family may have helped me to pause and feel the gravity of what I was doing. Something was needed to help me slow down for a moment to focus on Ma as a human being and my much-loved mother. I needed something tangible to remind me she was not just someone living in my home needing care. I needed to be mindful that what I was doing deserved to be done with effort and devotion.

I fell out of line, without the preemptive steps that should have been taken to remind me this was my mother for whom I was caring. I was prodded back into formation only by seeing Ma in some vulnerable pose or circumstance. The soft spot in my heart for Ma was never lost, only concealed by the daily work of caregiving.

Prayer helps many focus and trust that they are not alone when times are rough. I didn't have the correct disposition for quiet contemplation to reset my temperament. I was helped when I drew on the memory of Ma during my childhood, but it wasn't enough. Her history and her life were important to me. I needed more visual reminders of those memories, more quiet time to hold her hand and to be her son, not just a caregiver. The stress and duty of caregiving should not be allowed to fade or tarnish the memory of your loved one. Do all that you can to hang onto it.

Know your limits.

The capacity to give of oneself has a limit. Caring for more than you can may lead to stress, chronic pain, illness, depression, and anxiety. Responsibility that exceeds one's capability leads to poor attention to detail, mistakes, half-finished projects and compromised safety. We've all been there, feeling overwhelmed and paralyzed by excess work or responsibility. Knowing your limits takes more courage than trying to manage the unmanageable.

Caring for another human being is a special skill that not everyone can perform well for a day, much less months and years. It is a tough job, requiring an abundance of patience and physical strength. There is no fountain of eternal compassion that automatically refills the caregiver. One's ability to care must be nourished and replenished.

Anyone who feels overextended, stressed, spread too thin, or worn down needs to take a step back and reset before something "breaks." This is true in all circumstances but particularly important for caregivers. They are the pin that holds everything together. If they crack, everything changes for their loved one, themselves and the entire family. Caregivers must take care of themselves by knowing and understanding their own limits.

When approaching their limit, a caregiver must be humble enough to ask for help. Some appropriate and effective ways to reach out for help include family meetings, journaling, talking to a friend and writing notes to close family members. Other resources include doctors, nurses, therapists and church staff or fellow members.

People who are ready and willing to help are waiting to do so, but you need to let them know what you need. It is the responsibility of the caregiver to take the first step because unfortunately there may be no one around who knows what you do and what you need. Allow others the opportunity to help you.

Anticipate changes in the relationship with your loved one.

I was bewildered by what happened to the relationship between Ma and me. Was it the diaper changes, the demanding routines that caused the change? The ongoing, daily alteration of my life seemed to drain me of my good intentions. I resorted to a mechanical manner of caring that allowed me to get through my duties with little emotional energy spent.

Being a caregiver and a son at the same time was almost impossible. These two distinct types of social interaction couldn't easily coexist. One was uncomfortable work, requiring unpleasant activities such as contact with body fluids and messes to manage. The other was joyful and loving. There didn't seem to be enough time for the later and too much time required for the former. The impact was ominous.

The love I had for Ma was the immense, eternal love that is common between a parent and offspring. This natural love may seem to be enough fuel for long-lasting, compassionate caregiving, but it is not. All the work and challenges that come with caregiving impact the life of the caregiver and can dull the cutting edge of even the truest love. I began to wonder if it was beyond the natural human potential to care for another adult in such an all-encompassing way.

I wished I could have a simple, pleasant lunch with Ma and not have to deal with the mess and work that came with it. Taking the car and going to a drive-through was the closest I could come to perfection. Ma could eat a sandwich without too much difficulty, have a drink and we enjoyed some privacy not having to worry about others looking.

The totality of the emotions that accompanied the physical work left me exhausted. Not unlike other caregivers, my heart was saddened by the change in my relationship with the one I loved. When I warned others, who were about to care for their own parent, that their relationship would change, they looked at me quizzically, as if I had just told them the sun was square.

In certain ways, the relationship changes for the better. A newfound closeness may exist that had been missing before and the feeling of satisfaction that comes from being of help is fulfilling. The wishes and aspirations I had for caring for Ma came true in the first year and things were great. Then reality set in.

The strategy I needed and didn't have was to purposely make time to be her son. Five minutes of holding her hand, not needing to talk about anything would have been great. The changes are inevitable. Be aware and do what you must to be there for your parent as a son or daughter, not just a caregiver.

Understand your own emotions in the caregiving role.

It is human nature to coddle and protect a loved one in a time of illness or pain. The emotions of love and devotion are powerful motivators to step in and do whatever is needed for the health of the family member. This altruistic desire to help someone in need, especially a family member, is a highly desirable human characteristic.

The desire to comfort one's self when taking on the role of caregiver is also a strong force. The caregiver likely has some desire to have a noble purpose in life by providing for the needs of their family member. The desire to be wanted, needed and validated may provide motivation for the work. There are emotions of insecurity and fear about the eventual loss of the loved one, thus the caregiver naturally wants to prolong their life.

Just the desire to do what is right is itself a motivating factor. Most of us seeing an accident, or someone who has fallen, follow the instinct that urges us to help. If we instead walk away, we feel guilty.

However, the ability to be a caregiver is not in everyone. Living situations, including work and family, can prevent one from taking on this job. The typical caregiver is female, 50 years old, and responsible for 20 hours a week of caregiving work. It is usually the daughter of aging parents who takes on this role. Many caregivers must sacrifice their work careers to assist a parent. This level of self-giving for the betterment of another is not a capability all possess.

Stepping up to take care of an ailing loved one can save the rest of the family from many logistical and emotional decisions, worry and expense. Be aware of the many consequences that come with this big step and understand the most important and lasting motivation for this noble undertaking is love.

The care recipient's limitations in terms of pain, physical disability, emotional instability, or onset of dementia begin to impact the caregiver from the first day. The basic needs of the individual including meals, medication, toileting, bathing and dressing are all affected by whatever medical conditions are present. The most challenging conditions for a caregiver accompany dementia, Alzheimer's disease, and cancer.

When the honeymoon of caregiving is over things get tougher. For me, this was at the one-year mark. At this point, I began to feel the full impact of caregiving upon my life. The love for my mom never varied, but my fondness for doing what I thought was right did.

Feeling emotion is an important part of being human. The array of emotions encountered by caregivers include anger, boredom, anxiety, impatience, irritability, depression, sadness, disgust, frustration, guilt, grief, resentment, loss, jealousy, fatigue and burden. That sounds like an exhausting list and it is. There should be no shame when any of these emotions surface. The tendency may be to suppress and hide one's feeling for fear of appearing weak. That is a critical mistake.

Journaling is a way to express difficult thoughts and feelings the caregiver may never verbalize. This can be a very effective way to understand your own emotions. Re-reading entries in your journal can give you insight into which situations tend to cause more stress and provide you with motivation to make needed adjustments.

Just as pain is a warning sign of a physical problem, feelings of burden and depression should warn the caregiver to attend to their emotional health. Ignoring feelings will negatively affect the quality of the caregiver's life and compromise the care of the family member.

The spirit of the caregiver must be nourished, protected and kept healthy. It needs refreshing. One primary way to do that is to allow the caregiver to express their emotions. I believe caregivers are hesitant to be open about their feelings unless they are in the company of other caregivers who can relate to them without judgment. I have had caregivers pour their feelings out to me once they knew that I had been in a similar situation.

Caregiving support groups are available for certain diagnoses including stroke, spinal cord injury and Parkinson's Disease. Local hospitals and community centers may offer meetings for caregivers. The church community may offer home visits to those who have difficulty getting away from the house.

The roller coaster of emotion that a caregiver will feel is as real as your next breath. The ride is worse if you aren't allowed to scream! It is normal and healthy to express whatever emotions you feel. You only need one other person to hear you to make your life easier.

Absorb, don't react. Flex, don't break. Guide, don't force.

When the 'switch' flips, everything gets harder. Smooth waters become churning caldrons of unpredictable force. The 'switch' refers to the mental changes that can occur suddenly, primarily in those with Alzheimer's disease. The loved one's confusion, anger and depression can stretch an already overextended caregiver, and the timing of it is usually never good.

Caring for an elderly parent naturally gets harder as aging proceeds. Closer general supervision may be needed and tasks previously done independently may require assistance and guidance. These requirements to be at the patient's side more often lessen the caregiver's freedom. Less patience, a shorter temper, and an increased level of frustration are possible under these circumstances.

Take a deep breath. Walk away. Don't argue. If your loved one sees a cat crawling on the table, chase it away for them. If they see a box they want moved, move it. Reassure them in a calm tone of voice when they are afraid. Don't let their anxiety get the best of you.

They have no control over what is happening in their head and you can't change it either. Don't add fuel to the fire by forcing a certain response from them or trying to reason when they have no reasoning capability.

Figuratively, being poked in the eye while doing a good deed is part of being a caregiver. The extra 15 seconds it takes to do something because your loved one is not being cooperative may seem like an eternity, but it is not. The same bottle that opened easily every other day and is now suddenly stuck, is not behaving in such a manner just to annoy you. While you might tend to personalize such an event as a prank against your sanity, it certainly is not!

Find peace in whatever form you can. Know where your release valve is and use it regularly. Be smarter than your circumstances. Be cool and efficient. Less frustration will follow.

Be careful of what, when and how you say things, but say what needs to be said.

One of the rewards of caregiving is being close to your family member so that you can express words of love and appreciation regularly. This is especially true in cases of dementia or Alzheimer's disease where the window of opportunity tends to close over time. Unfortunately, the right mindset may not present itself nearly as often as you might hope during caregiving.

Choose the best time when the connection is the clearest and there is peace between you and your loved one. Take the time to sit together and listen to each other. Ask questions, hold each other's hands. These moments are golden nuggets that you can put in your pocket forever. They also fuel the fire of compassionate care. You never know how many of those opportunities you have left, and you cannot get back time lost after the passing of your loved one. Look for openings to take advantage of these precious moments. If you are rushed and in a hurry, they will slip by you.

More gets into the head of your loved one than you know. They hear, see and pay attention. Their face might not register what you say but don't be fooled. Agitated body language on your part can leave a horrible impression. Remember, the connections between their visual/communication centers and the origin of muscle activity for facial expression may be confused. A blank face doesn't necessarily mean no one is home. Respect this fact.

Do yourself a favor by knowing when to be quiet, when to refrain from reacting to inflammatory comments or situations. If you can master the art of suffering in silence, you will be much better off. Walk away for a moment. Come back when the air has cleared. Reacting with anger or in a negative way to some aberrant thought pattern expressed by your loved one is useless.

Reacting in anger can be dangerous and will only make the situation worse. The trick to being successful is to keep your pot from simmering beyond your own tolerance. This is a further illustration of the need for taking more breaks and providing respite care for yourself.

Seek out community contacts through church, support groups, friends, and neighbors.

Venturing out to make social contacts while working as a caregiver sounds like a daunting task when getting up in the morning can be hard enough. Cold calling on neighbors isn't necessary. The point is to take advantage of the resources in the community. There are those who are willing and able to help. There are many individuals who have this "silver lining" in their soul and want to help others. You just need to expend a little energy to find them.

For example, I wish I had been more insistent about Ma going to adult day care. I also isolated myself from the neighbors because of my own unwillingness to socialize. Even though I took Ma to church on several occasions I never took the opportunity to meet the many friendly, kind people there. I never considered attending a stroke survivor group. People want to help. You simply have to make yourself available for them to do so.

Why should you do any of these things? Because it takes just one individual to make your life so different and so much better. We as caregivers may shy away from socializing for our own selfish reasons. There is extra effort required to prepare two people to go out and face the public. You may have to explain, yet again, uncomfortable facts about your loved one's medical condition. Maybe you are just too exhausted to do anything beyond the bare essentials of a normal day. Possibly, but the enrichment and relief that can be provided by meeting one individual who is willing to help may be well worth the effort.

There is a self-conscious factor that may keep the caregiver from getting out into social settings. There may be a fear of uncooperative or badly timed bodily functions that you as caregiver need to deal with. Poor control of food or liquids may create messes requiring help, all while dealing with the stares of people who know no better. Most people, however, understand and will think nothing of it. You will be considered a star for what you do. No need for doubting thoughts.

Many caregivers do what they do in silence. There needs to come a time and place to open a window and let in fresh air. It is healthy for everyone involved to have social contact. It takes tilting just one domino to begin a chain reaction. Establishing help one time a week for an hour or two may reap rewards previously never thought of.

Make time for fun and entertainment.

Good soup needs to be stirred every now and then. In addition to all the other responsibilities a caregiver has, they are also in charge of entertainment. This is an important element for the sanity of both the caregiver and their loved one. Turning on the television doesn't count. Consider music, radio, games, art, hat day, singing, animals, fresh air plants, flowers, baking, etc. You can find almost every entertainment act ever recorded online at YouTube or Pandora.

The important thing is to create fun experiences to distract from the mundane, daily routines. Write a letter to an old friend. Read a short story or Hollywood gossip magazine, go for a drive. Plant an herb garden for the kitchen window. Activities outside the norm can ward off depression, stimulate the senses, and lighten the mood.

Enjoy chocolate sundaes, painting fingernails, memory games, exercising to a video, going for a walk. Do a jigsaw puzzle or do a crossword puzzle aloud. Idle minds wander, lose their attention span and become dull. The brain is like a muscle. The more you use it the stronger it remains.

Muscles benefit from being used at any age. Getting up and moving has countless rewards! Regular walks or wheelchair rides in the neighborhood are good for the physical being. They also set up the possibility of meeting a neighbor who might be willing to help. Senior exercise classes held at a local hospital or civic wellness center can serve the same purposes.

Doing things at the same time every day become incorporated into a routine much easier. This is especially true for exercise. A simple routine carried out to music or a program on television for only five minutes can benefit vitality. Simple arm movements, raising the hands overhead, doing sit-to-stands from a chair, or actively extending the knee with a point and flex of the foot are all beneficial things to do for anyone. If it is part of the daily routine you will tend to stick with it better.

A regularly scheduled radio program was one of my Ma's favorites. The radio is a wonderful device and it's free. Have a movie night, TV shows on DVD, or a coffee house date. Local churches and senior centers may offer programs at little to no cost.

Birthdays, holidays and anniversaries should be celebrated with glee. Using these events to separate one day from the next is important for the mental health of all involved. When you make your loved one feel special, above and beyond just being taken care of, your ability to care will be bolstered. Your efforts will come back to reward you, perhaps not the same day, but the rewards will come.

Preparing a favorite meal, a flower cut from the yard or a chocolate on the pillow at night are little things that make your loved one feel important and cherished, rather than a burden. A trip to the beauty parlor or barber, a manicure given by a grandchild, a visit over a cup of tea—these things will lift the spirits of everyone involved. These small things will require some forethought and planning but they are well worth the effort.

Having a corner set aside somewhere in the house to showcase family memories can be a source of pleasure for your loved one. This doesn't have to be anything more than a table or shelf with photos and knick- knacks, but it will have a wonderful effect on the brain of the one for whom you care. You may want to light a candle together to remember those who have passed. This activity can have a calming effect on your loved one and help them come to peace with their own mortality.

These types of activities can help rekindle the relationship between the caregiver and loved one which can lose its vitality during the caregiving process. Targeted, volitional effort needs to be aimed at keeping the fire lit. Never underestimate something as simple as baking cookies together when it comes to keeping good memories alive, maintaining a positive relationship and fueling your own compassion to continue to provide excellent care.

Let people know by sharing a journal or a letter with your honest thoughts. Have family meetings.

My journal helped me express my feelings, but it was a conversation I should have shared that I never did. Those who were closest to me would have been very surprised by what I said because I never let my burn-out show. Many caregivers feel they shoulder the load alone. They have anger toward other family members for not helping or at least acknowledging that the work being done is difficult.

Don't feel afraid to express feelings of burnout or burden. It's not a sign of weakness or an indication that you are unqualified for the job. You are not letting the family down. There is no need for shame. People won't know unless you say something, and they will likely be thankful when you do. Perhaps they always wanted to help but never knew how.

I propose journaling as a way of communicating with others. Journaling is an excellent way to capture the highs and lows when they are fresh in your mind. Sharing journal entries may be much easier than trying to verbally express what you are feeling. Fear of being embarrassed, judged or appearing weak may prevent the caregiver from expressing their true feelings. By presenting excerpts from a journal, in the form of a letter or note, the ice can be broken and any growing feelings of resentment or stress can be communicated without the need for an uncomfortable face to face meeting or phone call.

The goal is to create a dialogue with at least one other family member that will give them needed insight into the caregiving process. No one knows the full truth. No one gets it. And no one ever will unless steps are taken to let them know.

Regular family meetings are a great way to discuss issues. How the caregiver is getting along and handling all the obligations and responsibilities that face them should be a focus during the family meeting. Other family members can help by asking specific questions. "Tell us about the morning routine." "What are the primary challenges?" "What is the hardest part of the day?" "What can we do to help in any way?" "Are you getting enough time for yourself?"

The family meeting is the time for the caregiver to share their feelings, if not to the entire group gathered, then individually with the best candidate available. Use a written note to help crack the ice if that is easier, but the word must get out. This is the time, while the family is gathered, to address all concerns and issues. It may not happen again for another year. Don't miss your chance.

The loved one being cared for should also be allowed to express their feelings to the family without judgment. Let them talk. You listen. However, remember that certain conversations should take place outside their earshot. Respect their feelings by never allowing them to hear something said that they may interpret as their presence and condition being a burden to the rest of the family.

Outside caregivers should also be included in these meetings if possible to improve their accountability to and communication with the family.

Cherish yourself. You need it. You deserve it.

The importance of what a family caregiver does cannot be overstated. Not only do they assure the safety and health of a loved one, they also allow other family members to live their lives with little interruption. How fortunate are these other family members to have someone willing to step up and take on the role of caregiver!

This work requires sacrifices beyond what anyone else will ever see or fully appreciate. In terms of stress, both mental and physical and in terms of the magnitude of changes in the caregiver's life, the risk-reward ratio for this endeavor is "out of whack!" There is a National Caregiver Day, but it receives about as much attention as National Chewing Gum Day!

Caregivers need to look beyond the lack of acknowledgment they receive, and give themselves the credit they deserve for the noble job they do. They make the world a better place for their loved one and the entire family. Letting go of expectations for a pat on the back and affirmation of a job well done is a difficult, yet fruitful skill to learn. There will be no trophy for participation, no mention in the newspaper. The work of the caregiver is, however, no less important than that of a brain surgeon! They provide the life-giving care to a loved family member that many could not. Their reward is an inner peace that can endure forever.

Those with family members who appreciate the work being done are lucky and I have such a family. Although I felt they knew little of exactly what it took daily, I felt they were connected as best they could be, given the physical distance that separated us. Their knowledge of the daily realities was limited by geography and wasn't their fault, it was just the fact of the matter. I tried to keep them informed of the most important changes and events.

While external rewards are few, caregivers need to remind themselves of the less tangible, less obvious gifts they will receive. The closeness, memories, and struggles shared with their loved one all create a special place in the heart of the caregiver that others will never possess. The grief and sense of loss felt by the caregiver is a tribute to the sacrifices they made and the work they performed. This must be understood as reward and held onto as a lasting remembrance of a job well done.

SPIRITUAL HEALTH OF THE CAREGIVER

My siblings and I were not raised in a religious environment where we went to church on Sundays and prayed before each meal. Church services did not follow deaths of family members. Religion or prayers were not used in time of hardship for strength, or in good times to show gratitude. Personally, I was too cynical to accept the existence of God.

For these reasons, I do not feel qualified to talk about a higher power as a source of comfort for the caregiver. However, I fully appreciate and respect the importance of God in a person's life. Many caregivers I have talked to pray for the strength to continue. They pray to calm their souls and to lighten their load by handing it over to God.

During the care of my mom, especially in the last five years, my perceived burden and lack of a game plan left me out on a limb. What I needed, besides a coach, was an infusion of patience and serenity so I could see things, right in front of me, that may have helped. For example, the option of using adult day care for Ma as respite care for me was available but it never occurred to me. My eyes were open but I couldn't see. The humility I needed to put aside my own feelings for the sake of better care for Ma was absent. I needed internal peace to see the whole picture and I didn't have it.

I was not open enough to accept spiritual influence in my life, but I see now how it could have helped me. If I'd had an outlet for what I was feeling, a support group or person, or prayer that grounded me and eased my stress, I could have reacted better to challenging situations and maintained my ability to be compassionate.

Belief in a higher power comforts many in times of stress or loss. Prayer and connection to a religious community have been connected to living longer and healthier lives. While scientifically there may be a shortage of objective evidence to its specific effect, empirically speaking it cannot be challenged. Prayer helps!

There is no shame or guilt for not having been a regular church attendee or reader of the Bible and then later turning to God for strength and reassurance. Feelings of hypocrisy are unnecessary. There is no punishment for turning to God in time of need.

The diagnosis of cancer in an individual can draw them to call on God for help or blame Him for their illness. Sick or suffering people frequently want an answer to why this is happening to them. In the end, their goal is to find peace. Spirituality is a source of peace for many.

Toward the end of my mom's life, she indicated interest in going to church or seeing a priest, when there had been no such interest in the past. Ma may have had an inner desire to connect spiritually. After her mini-stroke, she prayed with Nikki, my ex-wife. No one before had ever attempted to do this with Ma. I didn't know she had this desire.

When the chaplain started coming as part of hospice service, Ma seemed to perk up with her arrival. They talked about things, maybe nothing specific in relation to God, but the presence of this chaplain made a difference for my mom.

The American Academy of Family Physicians medical information website at https://familydoctor.org/spirituality-and-health/ defines spirituality as, "the way you find meaning, hope, comfort and inner peace in your life." No reference to God or a higher power is made. Peace may come in the form of a Yoga class, a walk around the yard, or sitting in a special corner of the house meditating. For those who wish to turn to God, there is no timetable, designated hours of operation, or need for a special pass to talk with Him. He is available 24/7.

Having faith in the belief that God is at your side can certainly be a virtue when you are a caregiver. Coming to this point of faith may require soul searching, and shredding of previously ingrained beliefs and prejudices, but for those who have done so the rewards can be significant. Accepting God's plan and relinquishing anger towards enemies and events that have caused great stress is considered to be healthy. Prayer, rituals, church, quiet space and time for talking to God or reading the Bible are ways to find peace.

Dr. Carol Peters-Tanksley is a contributor to the website *The Caregivers Voice*, a valuable source of information for caregivers. Dr. Carol is an OB-Gyn physician, Doctor of Ministry, author and speaker. She also was a caregiver for her husband Al. Dr. Carol brings firsthand knowledge of the physical, emotional and spiritual demands of caring for a loved one.

She speaks of three spiritual-life tips that helped her through what she describes as exhaustive work in helping her husband prior to his death. These include regular soul nourishment, reassurance of the future, and perspective and purpose. Dr. Carol used prayer and teachings from the Bible to provide strength on her journey with her husband.

Regular Soul Nourishment

It is critically important for the spirit of the caregiver to remain loving and compassionate. It must be bolstered and replenished. This can be accomplished through meditation, quiet alone-time and 'time outs' from the caregiving work. Contact with the church community through home visits can be beneficial. A few minutes of prayer a day is described by Dr. Carol as "water for a person dying of thirst."

This concept of filling the empty tank, if you will, has been described in other walks of life as an analogy to providing the needed "stoking of the fire" to achieve revival of the spirit. Business management seminars use this idea in motivating and empowering employees. Marriage counselors practice this as a way of bringing two people together again after a fallout or marital turmoil. The same concept holds true for caregivers to remain compassionate in the care they provide. You cannot keep withdrawing from an account unless you also make deposits. Just as employees need motivation and couples need understanding and mutual respect, the caregiver needs a refreshed and revitalized spirit. It's very difficult to remain loving and motivated to give compassionate care when you feel you can't go on much longer.

Reassurance of the Future

Issues of guilt, resentment and regret powerfully influence emotion and behavior. They can pull a caregiver down and deplete their ability to love. Many thoughts repeated themselves in my head during my years with Ma. I worried about what I was giving up in life. I wondered how much longer I could go on caring for Ma as I was. I was changing as a person but was mostly unaware of the changes. Evidence of this was my growing belief that I could not and would not ever let my own kids take care of me in this way.

Fearing the loss of a family member can be an additional weight to bear, while simultaneously caring for the person. Providing care can draw you closer to them and make it harder to let go when they pass. And what will your purpose be once that family member is gone? The meaning and importance of rising each new day may be lost.

In the Bible, God assures that you are not given more than you can handle and that He is at your side always. You are taught that your life matters and that your future is in God's hands. Encouragement is given to realize that there are spiritual powers in control greater than you, and that peace is promised.

Direction and purpose may become lost when the tunnel is dark. We all want light. Prayer and belief may help the caregiver who feels lost and alone.

Perspective and Purpose

I've related extensively how I lost my perspective and my tether to what was my most important goal for Ma, that she would receive compassionate loving care all the way to the end. This was clearly stamped on my mind and heart in the beginning. But the burdens of caregiving became too heavy for me. I could not do it alone without a strategy and tools to allow me to stay firm in my conviction.

Those who put their faith in a higher power are not alone. They can believe God has chosen them for the duty of caring for another human being. In this, caregivers can take strength from being entrusted with such an important responsibility. The daily work required can be considered a reminder of God's will. Talking to God in prayer and about this is a very personal experience, and a source of peace that accompanies the responsibility that the caregiver bears.

Stress comes from lacking control in a situation or set of circumstances and caregivers often feel out of control. However, feeling a sense of purpose, rising to challenges and finding peace through it all is possible when keeping the correct perspective about what you are doing and for whom you are doing it. Faith in a higher power can help the caregiver keep this perspective.

Starting and ending each day with peacefulness in prayer can set the emotional tone for what's ahead. Meditation, prayer, and journaling can be ways of expressing normal emotions that the caregiver may be hesitant to display otherwise. Ill emotions fester when held in. Surrendering control to God, expressing feelings, receiving rest and renewal of the spirit are hallmarks of spiritual wellness in the caregiver.

I am certainly not an authority in this field, but if I'd had a source of humbleness and strength, my vision would have been better. Things would have been done differently. A caregiver's health can certainly benefit from their belief in a higher power.

STATISTICS OF CAREGIVERS IN THE UNITED STATES

The National Alliance for Caregiving and the AARP Public Policy Institute published <u>Caregiving in the U.S. 2015</u>, a study detailing the needs and feelings of unpaid caregivers. Previous studies were conducted in 1997, 2004 and 2009. This valuable information paints a portrait of family caregivers in America today. It is based on online interviews of 1,248 unpaid caregivers, age 18 and older who provide care to an adult.

Key elements of the study included the following:

*The prevalence of caregivers in the U.S.
*Demographic characteristics of caregivers and care recipients.

*The caregiver's situation in terms of the nature of caregiving activities, the intensity and duration of care, the health conditions and living situation of the person to whom care is provided, and other unpaid and paid help provided.

*How caregiving affects caregiver stress, strain, and health.

*Information needs related to caregiving.

*Public policy and caregiver support.

In this study, special attention for need identification is given to groups of caregivers who face complex, high-burden care situations resulting in higher stress and strain for them. These groups include older caregivers, caregivers who had no choice in taking on their caregiving role, and the higher hour caregivers (those providing more than 21 hours per week of caregiving.)

A summary document of Caregiving in the U.S., 2015 can be obtained through The National Alliance of Caregiving at www.caregiving.org

The following are excerpts from this invaluable document. Every attempt is made to keep these statistics with the original context of the document.

*43.5 million adults or 18.2% of the U.S. population age 18 or older have provided unpaid care to adults or children in the year prior to the survey.

*34.2 million adults or 14.3% of the U.S. population have provided care to an adult age 50 or older in this same period.

*60% of all caregivers are female; 40% are male.

*The average caregiver is 49 years old.

*One out of ten caregivers are 75 years old or older. The average within this group is represented by a 79-year-old female caring for a 77-year-old male, at least 34 hours a week. She has been providing this care for 5.6 years and deals with Alzheimer's disease, 'old age issues', and heart disease. Forty-six percent of this group report a high burden of care with the following issues providing the most stress: communicating with healthcare professionals, advocating for care and managing finances (usually on a fixed income).

*85% of unpaid caregivers care for a family member.

*49% are caring for a parent or parent-in-law.

*10% are caring for a spouse.

*Eight out of ten caregivers are caring for one person.

*Average length of caregiving service currently being provided is 4 years.

*The typical recipient of care is a female 69.4 years of age.

*More than half of all care recipients have been hospitalized in the past 12 months.

*59% of care recipients suffer a long-term physical condition, 35% a short-term physical condition and 26% have memory problems. 37% of recipients have more than one ongoing problem.

*Nearly half of all caregivers provide care to someone 75 years or older.

*Half of all recipients receive care in their own home.

*Higher hour caregivers (those providing care at least 21 hours a week) are more likely to live with their care recipient.

*The average caregiver provides 24.4 hours a week of care.

*23% of caregivers provide care more than 41 hours a week.

*The average higher hour caregiver is 52 years old and has been providing care for 5.6 years.

*The following are six activities of daily living assisted by caregivers and the percentage of caregivers who assist with each task:

> Getting in and out of bed and chairs 43%
> Getting dressed 32%
> Getting to and from the toilet 27%

Bathing and showering 26%
Feeding 23%
Dealing with incontinence and diapers 16%

*The most difficult activities of daily living involve personal care activities such as dealing with incontinence and diapers, helping the recipient to and from the toilet, and bathing/showering assistance.

*Instrumental Activities of Daily Living include the following with the percentage of caregivers who help with each activity:

Transportation 78%
Grocery or other shopping 76%
Housework 72%
Preparing meals 61%
Managing finances 54%
Giving medications, pills or injections 46%
Arranging for outside services 31%

*Six out of ten caregivers assist with 'medical nursing tasks' which include injections, tube feedings, and colostomy care. Just 14% of those who assist with these activities report having received some preparation or training to perform these tasks.

*32% of all family caregivers state their loved one gets paid help from homecare aides, housekeepers, agencies or others. One in three caregivers have no help at all, either paid or unpaid.

*Caregivers who had no choice in taking on the role of caring for a loved one report higher stress and strain levels and more complex care situations. This group is especially likely to report a negative impact on their life because of providing care.

*One in five caregivers report high levels of physical strain from caregiving. Two in five consider caregiving to be emotionally stressful.

*Caregivers who deal with chronic or long term conditions are particularly prone to emotional stress. About one half of all caregivers report feeling emotionally stressed when caring for someone with a mental health issue such as Alzheimer's disease or dementia, or any long term physical condition.

*Six in ten caregivers report being unemployed at some point in the past year while caregiving. The impact of work combined with caregiving causes 6 out of 10 caregivers to make a workplace accommodation such as cutting back hours, or talking a leave of absence.

*More than 8 out of 10 caregivers state they could use more information or help on caregiving topics. Caregivers most commonly want information on keeping their loved one safe at home, managing their own stress, managing challenging behaviors and dealing with incontinence or toileting issues.

Unpaid caregivers are an integral part of the formal health care, long-term services and support systems for the aging population. In the summary of the 2015 study, the following key areas were noted to need attention:

*Identify and help caregivers who are at risk of deteriorating health, financial insecurity and decreased quality of life.

*Identify and advocate for programs that could make a real difference in caregivers' well-being and in their ability to continue providing care, including helping them balance paid employment and unpaid care.

*Give caregivers resources to cope with the sometimes unexpected and sudden entry into providing care.

*Extend training to caregivers who perform ADLS (Activities of Daily Living Services), medical/nursing tasks, and other activities, including communicating and interacting with the formal care system.

*Encourage families to proactively plan for and discuss aging and health/disability. Include planning for the future and scenarios where the current unpaid caregiver may no longer be able to provide care.

RESPITE CARE

Respite care is the single most important factor for the health of a caregiver. The quality of care received by the family member may depend most on whether the caregiver is allowed a regular consistent break from caregiving work. The spirit of the caregiver is like gold and must be treated as such.

The definition of respite is a short period of rest or relief from something difficult or unpleasant. Respite care is temporary care given to persons with disabilities or special health care needs, providing relief for their usual caregiver.

My career was my only respite care during the ten years of caring for my mother. This was a big mistake. I needed more leisure time to take care of myself and only myself.

A hired caregiver took care of Ma while I was at work and that gave me peace of mind to know that Ma was being cared for during my time away. I was supposed to be home between six and six thirty to relieve the paid caregiver. She didn't want to leave Ma alone, so if I was late, she would frequently stay. I felt pressure to get home on time. Once home I would get dinner for Ma if she hadn't yet eaten. I would ask her how her day was and then a pressure inside me began to build and I would feel compelled to leave.

I couldn't stay in the house after I'd assured Ma was fed and had something to drink. I would put Ma in her recliner where she would be safe and then I'd make an excuse to leave for an hour or two. I'd have dinner with Darlene, or I would aimlessly go to the store to buy something not necessarily needed, just so I wouldn't have to be there on caregiver duty.

Some days were different. Some days I'd sit exhausted on the couch with Ma eight feet in front and to the right of me in her recliner. There would be no communication, just a brainless TV lighting up the room for 3 to 4 hours before bed. Sometimes I would retire to my room leaving Ma alone in the living room to stare blankly at the screen. I would check on her every now and then but I was exhausted and out of energy for caring.

While I was away from Ma, during the day at work, I was listening to people, solving problems and giving of myself. When I picked up the caregiving torch at home, it was too heavy for me. I had to get out of the house to save my sanity. My ability to always be an attentive son was impaired.

When the weekends came, it was all on me from Friday night to Monday morning. There were chores to do, errands to run, maintenance tasks to perform around the house in addition to the meals, diaper changes, bathing and dressing for Ma. By Sunday night, going back to work felt like a vacation.

I needed time for myself. There was no time available to be away both from Ma and work so I could do the things I wanted to do for myself. Instead, I took chances by leaving Ma alone so I could have a short break.

My batteries for caregiving would recharge partially while I was at work, but there was a slow steady drain occurring which eventually affected my compassion. I never arranged for a regular schedule of respite care, 2-5 hours a week, when I could go and do what I wanted to without worry that Ma would get into trouble or need my help.

There were several factors preventing me from seeking respite care. The first, and prominent one was not perceiving the need for it. I knew something was happening inside of me. What else could explain my swings in temperament. There was litmus test for burnout, and I wasn't about to openly complain. Thus, no diagnosis and no treatment plan. This led me down an unhealthy path for that of a caregiver.

Money was a definite factor, as paid caregivers are expensive. The money that was coming in covered the caregiving needs Monday through Friday with no extra remaining for respite care. If I could do it over, I'd ask for 4 hours a week of paid respite care from my siblings. They didn't know the need, and I can't blame them because I never said anything. But that's what I should have done.

Availability was another factor. I was not one to reach out for help. I did not seek connections with neighbors or church or local organizations to help me. Something about imposing on others, combined with Ma's fear of having someone else handle her, if needed, during a transfer to the toilet prevented me from seeking additional help.

Finding a neighbor to sit with Ma could have been possible, but I never tried. My kids were busy with their own lives and I didn't want to depend on them. I felt uncomfortable leaving others to deal with Ma's drool problems and bathroom needs.

In hindsight, I should have simply done it. It would have worked out. We were all adults and accommodations for Ma's needs in my absence could have been made. I should have stepped outside my comfort zone and advertised for a sitter by way of a neighborhood flyer or word of mouth. Good, caring people step forward in time of need. This would have been good for Ma socially and provided her with added stimulation.

The local church community could have been a source of help. We didn't need to be religious or regular church attendees to receive some sort of volunteer help. But I never even thought to ask for someone else to research this resource for me.

Adult day care was never on my radar screen as a source of respite care. Even after I visited a facility, I didn't consider it. Ma refused to attend for the benefits of socialization and stimulation for herself, but I should have been more insistent. This facility was very clean with helpful staff and fun activities available. Ma needed help to the bathroom, which they did not provide, but she wore a diaper and the risk/reward ratio favored considering this as a method of respite care.

Professional sources of respite services include caregiving agencies, home health services and hospice care (if qualified). These avenues of care can be researched through the internet. Research shows that only 12% of caregivers utilize the internet on a regular basis. The responsibility for an internet search should be taken on by other family members who have the time and capability. Internet searches should include local hospitals, county social services and organizations such as The American Red Cross, AARP and websites such as the Family Care Alliance and Respite Care-Eldercare Locator. See the reference section at the end of this book. See the reference section for further options.

The caregiver's pride tends to run deep. While providing loving care may be their strong suit, asking for help may be their downfall. Caregivers will tend to hide their feelings and plod ahead instead of seeking assistance.

Caregiving work demands that the caregiver stand up for themselves. If phone calls and family meetings don't appeal to the caregiver, then a written form of communication can be effective. Writing a letter explaining your need for some time for yourself may open a world previously unknown.

Send up a flare! Ask for help. This is not a sign of weakness.

You can advertise for help in local newspapers, on job boards, or in internet services like Craig's list or Angie's list. We used Craig's lit to locate our caregivers and had only success. We interviewed applicants with Ma present and checked references. We found some potential caregivers that asked for a minimum number of hours. Many have more than one client and to maximize the efficiency of their schedule they require a minimum of 10 hours a week. There are a lot of good people out there looking for steady work. Be cautious, be picky and trust your gut.

It's impossible to talk about respite care without also talking about money. There are programs that will pay caregivers for the assistance they provide their own family members. There are some qualifications and the pay is at minimum wage, but there are many caregivers who can qualify for these programs. For more information about such programs, contact County social services.

In my first example of caring, James and his wife take care of their autistic sons. They receive respite care through a county program that benefits families caring for children with autism or Down's Syndrome. James says that this has been a lifesaver for him and his wife because, as he puts it, "It's hard to be loving and caring when you are stressed all the time."

You can't expect help for free. If other family members are unwilling or unable to assist physically with care, maybe they could help financially. Paying for a sitter or healthcare aide for several hours a week would be of great help.

Family caregivers may feel a financial squeeze if they have to cut their hours at work to do what they need to at home. Some have to quit their jobs altogether. If caregivers are lucky enough to realize they need respite care, they often pay for it themselves, deepening an already existing hardship. This amplifies the need to request help from outside family members.

Personal needs and responsibilities, health and well-being tend to reside near the bottom of a caregiver's totem pole. The energy to deal with self-maintenance simply isn't there much of the time. If caregivers can't get away from their caregiving work, they may never see the need to take care of themselves just as well as they care for others.

The health of the caregiver and care recipient depends on time away from caregiving work for the caregiver. A candle doesn't last forever and burns out even faster when burning at both ends. This can easily happen to the caregiver. Respite care is the single most important factor to maintain the loving and giving spirit of the caregiver.

ALZHEIMER'S DISEASE

Dementia is the general term used to describe memory disorders, personality changes, and impaired reasoning. Alzheimers disease is the most common cause of dementia in those over 65 years of age. Other causes of dementia include infections, metabolic disorders, nutritional deficiencies, or reaction to a head injury.

Alzheimer's disease is diagnosed in several ways. There are relatively easy cognitive/problem questions or tests administered by a physician during a regular doctor visit. There is also the MRI (Magnetic Resonance Imaging) which reveals the existence of plaques or opaque areas of the brain in the Alzheimer's patient. Usually, however, the simple questioning and physical exam of the patient is enough to confirm the diagnosis.

The cause of Alzheimer's disease is unknown. There may be a combination of genetic, lifestyle and environmental factors involved in its occurrence. Scientists have discussed the build-up of two abnormal compounds called *amyloid plaques* and *neurofibrillary tangles* in association with Alzheimer's disease. Age-related changes in the brain may cause atrophy of certain parts of the brain and its neurons, which are the pathways on which messages travel through the brain, contributing to the disorder.

Most patients with Alzheimer's disease have the type termed 'late-onset', with symptoms becoming apparent in their mid 60's. Early-onset Alzheimer's disease seems to have a strong genetic factor with symptoms occurring between the ages of 30 and 60.

The following symptoms in those diagnosed with Alzheimer's disease reflect the changes in cognitive (mental processing) capabilities:

* memory loss, especially short term (events occurring as recently as yesterday)

* difficulty communicating or finding words

* difficulty with reasoning and problem solving

* difficulty handling complex tasks, such as following 2 and 3 step directions

* difficulty with planning and organization

* difficulty with coordinated motor function

* confusion/disorientation

Motor control issues and impaired judgement create risk for injury from falls and dangerous activities attempted during a state of confusion. There may be the tendency to wander off, necessitating the need for constant supervision. Measures must be taken to secure doors with locks and alarms.

The psychological effects of Alzheimer's disease can include the following:

* personality changes

* depression

* anxiety

* inappropriate behavior

* paranoia

* agitation

* hallucinations

The above-mentioned deficits can occur individually or in combination. They can be transient, increasing in frequency and intensity, without cause or apparent reason. Cycles of good days and bad days can repeat themselves for years during a slow gradual decline in overall function.

Deterioration of independent function, self-care, ambulation and daily activities increases the physical demand on the caregiver. The patience of the caregiver can be challenged to its limit when the loved one's confusion overtakes their ability to reason.

Caregivers refer to this as the 'switch.' When the Alzheimer's patient goes from docile and coherent to confused and belligerent, it's as if a switch has been flipped. This sudden change in behavior causes the most stress for the caregiver of an Alzheimer's patient.

Tasks that require close physical contact between the two parties can become violent interactions. Caregivers may be slapped, pushed or sucker-punched. Threats of physical harm from the care recipient to the caregiver are not unusual.

Violent behavior and verbal attacks can't be taken lightly, and the caregiver's resolve and desire to continue in their role will be put to the test. To handle these events the caregiver must have the correct mindset and level of patience. A caregiver who attempts to force their will upon an agitated Alzheimer's patient will likely only make things worse.

Meal times can also be particularly challenging as the care recipient's appetite decreases and their chewing and swallowing abilities decline. The loved one may think their caregiver is trying to hurt them during times of feeding. Feelings of failure and frustration are natural on the part of the caregiver in this scenario and mounting tension on both sides can be a recipe for physical and verbal confrontations.

Changing clothes and bathing require proximity between the one assisting and the one being assisted, presenting the potential for the Alzheimer's patient to be more agitated. Any situation where the Alzheimer's patient becomes frightened or disoriented can compromise the safety of both parties. It is essential for the caregiver to have the proper mindset to manage these situations.

A caregiver cannot force. They must take what is given, and present guidance. There is no need to fight; it is important to maintain a peaceful atmosphere. There is no making sense of nonsense, so reasoning is not indicated. An angry caregiver should walk away.

It is important to realize that insults or threats are not personal. They are the result of abnormally firing neurons in the complex human brain. The Alzheimer's patient is an unwilling victim of their disease.

It is critical to create a safe, comfortable and efficient environment for both the caregiver and care recipient. Organize the bathroom, dressing and feeding areas so that everything needed is close at hand. The diaper supply should not be in the next room. Wipes must be immediately available when needed. All medications should be kept in one place. The feeding area should be easy to access for both people and close to cups, straws, napkins and silverware. Properly placed grab bars, assistive devices for ambulation (walkers, gait belts) and a clear path, free of obstacles are all essential to avoid the risk of tripping or falling.

Timing and pacing of activity are vitally important. Choose time during the day when the 'switch' is in the desirable direction, when things are calm to do tasks like bathing or others that require communication and closeness. A calm approach and soft guidance when requesting an action can defer an altercation. Gentle gets it done. Force leads to failure.

There is a Spanish phrase I tried to keep in mind while caring for my mom. "Sigue la corriente," means "go with the flow." That is an excellent policy to follow when caring for someone with Alzheimer's disease.

THE DYING PROCESS

Sudden death leaves a void that is difficult to comprehend. Life has changed permanently in a fleeting moment. Never being able to say the things that you need or desire to say may leave a horrible pain and sense of loss. Like the healing of a wound, time is needed to make a proper adjustment to this life changing event.

A prolonged death means watching life slowly extinguish itself. Feeling out of control and helpless to assist in a meaningful way may tear at one's heartstrings. Contemplating the comparison of the healthy, premorbid state of the individual to their current physical condition may be too much to bear.

The dying process subjects the survivors to a vast array of emotions. There is no manual to tell us exactly how we should react or feel. The obvious answers are sadness, sorrow, depression, anger, and relief. Though the sense of loss may be deep, hopefully there also a feeling of peace that pain and suffering have ended, and the spirit is now free.

The turn toward death and the beginning of grieving can occur long before the last breath. My mom's TIA, or mini-stroke, occurring eight months before her death was the beginning of the end for her, although I did not recognize it at the time. There were subtle signs; decreased alertness, increased sleepiness, less appetite and poor fluid manipulation. The work required of me to care for her increased, but the thought of death didn't enter my mind, even after she told us, "This is the end of life."

She was frail, but the compassion of my care did not always follow in step with her frailty. Burnout, denial, fear, the work of caregiving, my lack of knowledge about dying all went hand in hand toward my absence of appreciation that she was steering toward death. Eight months later she was gone.

Ma's bravery and tolerance are etched in my memory. In countless ways, I was lucky. Many caregivers deal with much more than I did. Ma was never angry, verbally abusive or physically abusive. She didn't wander. For those caregivers who have had to deal with such behaviors from their loved one, while providing care as death approached, I can only pass on my respect and admiration.

I requested hospice care for my mom after the TIA, not because I knew she was dying, but because I wanted her monitored more closely than I could provide. A nurse came to examine Ma two to three days a week. Pulse, blood pressure and breathing were checked. Ma, on a good day, would have conversation with them. Peace of mind was the bonus for me. Between hospice and the paid caregiver, Paula, Ma was taken care of well.

Meanwhile, the signs were present that things were changing for the worse. The report I'd frequently receive from the caregiver told me Ma's appetite was poor and she was sleeping most of the day. When I returned home, Ma usually would awaken for at least a short while before falling asleep again. She often had a few great days, being alert and eating well. Then she would regress back into a passive, lethargic state that would sometimes require I physically had to lift her from chair to chair. Previously she had assisted me with all her might.

The indications of approaching death do not have a predictable, chronological order and are not consistent from case to case. Variances can depend on the overall health of the individual and their organ system, along with age, diagnosis, medications used and the presence of family support.

There are two phases in the dying process, known as the "pre-active phase of dying" and the "active phase of dying." The pre-active phase lasts up to two weeks but can be longer, up to 6 to 8 weeks. The active phase of dying usually lasts 3 to 4 days, but can extend, up to one to two weeks. There can be transitions between these two phases.

The pre-active phase is characterized by the following:

*inordinate weakness and fatigue

*bed-bound status in formerly active patients

*increased sleep

*progressive disorientation

*limited attention span

*restlessness

*decreased interest in food and liquid

*difficulty swallowing

*loss of bowel and bladder control

*need for oxygen

*increased dependence on caregivers to provide basic needs

Transition into the active phase of dying occurs when oxygenation to the organ systems of the body is compromised and these systems of the kidneys, liver, heart and lungs begin to shut down.

The active phase of dying includes the following characteristics:

*decreased responsiveness

*eyes glassy, pupils unfocused

*no interest in food or water

*cessation of urination

*lowered blood pressure

*abnormal respiratory pattern

*blood pressure and pulse difficult to obtain

*progressive cooling and mottling of extremities

*excess secretions and congestion

*lowered skin temperature (skin cool, clammy, damp)

*nail beds and mucous membranes begin to turn purple

The day following the incident in the bathroom with my mom, hospice came to the house and declared that Ma's care should now be palliative, with efforts now being directed for comfort and not sustainability. Everything concerning Ma's care changed. Arrangements were made in the house to locate her bed for easy access by healthcare providers and family during the progression of her final days.

Most importantly, the decision was made to withhold food and fluid, partly to avoid possible aspiration or choking, but also to comfortably end her life. I second guessed this decision in my mind, feeling I should have fought for more time. Ma's breathing pattern and level of responsiveness changed dramatically after that night in the bathroom. She was extremely weak and fatigued, but she had pulled through similar situations before. We assumed she had suffered another stroke. She was home with family and comfortable. Was this what she would want? We kept vigil at Ma's bedside.

Her only intake orally was morphine, to slow her respirations when they became labored or too rapid. We talked to her, held her hand, combed her hair. We know she heard and felt our presence.

Hospice care is a wonderful service that should be requested when a family member is being cared for at home. The request must be made to the patient's primary care doctor. Services provided by hospice include visits from a nurse and social worker. Nurse's aides assist with bathing and dressing which can be of great help to the family caregiver.

Many hospice services also have volunteers who will assist with some of the daily duties around the house, depending on the needs of the care recipient. Chaplain visits can provide a great deal of comfort. The information hospice provides about the dying process is invaluable. If hospice is not offered, ask about it. You and your loved one are entitled to this service during the end of life months and the benefits are immense.

CEREBRAL VASCULAR ACCIDENT (CVA OR STROKE)

The ramifications of a stroke can be significant for the victim and their family. Strokes occur in the brain where the neural pathways traverse from one side of the brain to the other. A stroke on the right side of the brain will affect the left side of the body and vice-versa. Communication ability, judgment, and personality can be altered, depending on where in the brain a stroke occurs.

Per the Center for Disease Control, cerebral vascular accident (CVA), or stroke, accounts for 1 out of every 20 deaths. Someone in the U.S. has a stroke every 45 seconds. Every year, more than 795,000 people in the U.S. suffer a stroke.

Nearly three-quarters of all strokes occur in people over the age of 54, although they can occur at any age. The risk of stroke doubles each decade after the age of 55. Having one stroke does not necessarily mean you will have another.

Strokes are caused by an interruption in the blood supply to a portion of the brain, either by blockage (87% of all strokes) or hemorrhage. Hemorrhagic strokes can cause more damage than ischemic strokes (those caused by a blockage). The resulting deficits of a stroke depend on where in the brain the stroke occurred. Strokes can vary from very mild to severe. Hypertension (high blood pressure) is the main risk factor for stroke.

The initial symptom of a stroke is typically numbness on one side of the body or face. An altered level of consciousness or a period of confusion may also be present along with slowed or slurred speech.

Emergency medical services are needed as quickly as possible when these initial symptoms appear. Patients who arrive at the emergency room within 3 hours of their first symptoms often have less disability three months after their stroke, compared to those who receive delayed care.

If the symptoms subside within 30 minutes, a TIA (or trans ischemic attack), also referred to as a 'mini-stroke,' may have occurred. A brief period of confusion, slurred speech or lack of mobility can indicate a TIA.

When initial symptoms do not subside, hospitalization is required for monitoring and stabilization of the patient, followed by rehabilitation. Recovery can be rapid in some cases, with little residual effect. Age, pre-existing medical conditions and the severity of the interruption in blood flow will determine the outcome.

After a stroke, as swelling and inflammation in the brain subside, healing begins. The brain has tremendous healing power allowing for function to begin to return. Slowly, cognition and speech may return to normal. Most of the improvement following a stroke will occur in the first six months.

Severe strokes can deprive a person of physical and communicative ability, while minor strokes may result in a lazy hand and a weak foot on the involved side, without severe functional deficits. Everything depends on the extent of the damage and the location in the brain where it occurred.

There are many who have suffered strokes who function well and live independently. Others require assistance from a caregiver or family member for bathing, dressing, and self-care. A stroke survivor may be able to stand and pivot to transfer by themselves to a chair or toilet, but not be able to ambulate without a cane. If walking is unsafe, risking a fall, a wheelchair may be necessary for mobility around the home and in the community. This may be a temporary need until further strength and balance return.

The left side of the brain controls the right side of the body and vice versa. Stroke on the left side of the brain will affect the right side of the body and stroke on the right side of the brain will affect the left side of the body, changing muscle tone, strength, and control. There can be changes on both sides of the body with a very severe stroke, but typically they are confined to just one side.

The hand and foot are most significantly impaired due to their large representation on the cerebral cortex where movements are initiated. Losing function of one hand is not unusual in a moderate to severe stroke. The foot may drag while walking, or the knee may become unstable. There are many ways to manage these weaknesses.

When the trunk is affected, there will be difficulty with upright sitting and balance. Problems with balance create a risk for fall necessitating close supervision by another when the stroke victim sits on the edge of the bed or attempts to stand from a sitting position. Assistance will be needed to transfer between different seating surfaces.

Sensory changes can take place which interfere with one's ability to detect the position of the arm or leg in space. This is called proprioception and is an important ability for personal care and walking. The stroke victim may become spatially unaware of their affected side, causing them to bump into doorways or to travel close to the wall on one side or the other.

Visual and sensory deficits complicate the motor and strength impairment in a stroke patient. Compensatory strategies and movement are learned in therapy to help mitigate these deficits. Time will tell as to how much these sensory deficits subside.

The speech center is located on the left side of the brain in 80% of the population. Strokes in the left side of the brain, therefore, can often impair the ability to express or understand the spoken word, making the ability to formulate sentences, and process or interpret commands, difficult. Speech therapy should be sought early on to address these conditions.

Emotional instability and impaired judgment may occur, depending on the site of involvement. These changes can pose serious demands on the person caring for the stroke victim. Education for the caregiver and family explaining the source of these changes will increase their understanding of the behaviors that can be exhibited.

Depression can occur in a stroke victim when they see their function failing to return. Having to rely on someone else to do the things for them they could once do on their own is disheartening. It is important to reassure them that they are loved and, although their physical being is impaired, the core of who they are remains intact. One day at a time, one step at a time, everything will be alright.

Physical, Occupational, and Speech Therapy are used to facilitate improvement in the stroke patient. These services can be received both on an inpatient and outpatient basis and usually begin from day one in the hospital. If improvements are ongoing, these services can continue. Good family support and help will further the rehabilitation process once formal therapy has stopped.

Family members who care for the stroke victim need to be educated on proper techniques for moving the patient, to assure the safety of the patient and themselves, avoiding injuries to both. Wheelchairs, grab bars, commodes, and walking aids may be needed to assist with mobility. Education regarding these matters must be requested from the doctor and local rehabilitation departments. Support groups for the victims and families affected by stroke are available in most communities through a local hospital or the National Stroke Association.

EPILOGUE

It has been eighteen months since my mom passed. Just yesterday I took several truckloads of junk to the local landfill. Included was my mom's wheelchair which was too old and worn to donate. I left it there in the dirt, standing up, leg rests attached and then I drove away, saddened, thinking of Ma sitting in that chair. I made two more trips to the dump over the next few hours. On the second trip, I could still see my mom's chair but not on the third trip. I visually scanned but couldn't find it so, just before leaving, I waded through the rubbish to get near the area where I'd left it. I wanted to see it, feel it one last time.

Finally, the handles appeared through an opening between an upside-down couch and something else, I don't remember what. I put my hands on the armrest of that chair and looked down into it as if she were still there. Letting go of that chair yesterday was tough. Do I still have a way to go? Yes, I do. But that is what caring for someone you love does.

I am humbled by this ten-year experience with my mom. I thought I had it handled, but I didn't. Ma knew of my stress and tried to make things as easy as possible for me. Her strength and tolerance were astounding. She will never know the lessons she taught and I am indebted to her forever.

Writing this book helped lessen my grief after my mom passed. However, its real purpose and message are for the caregiver: Stay on the beam. Your loved one's welfare and the serenity of your soul depend on it. A preemptive strike against the volatile mixture of caregiving and the needs of your own life is necessary to assure the proper care of your loved one.

Taking on the responsibility of being a caregiver often occurs at an inconvenient time in life. Career work, raising children or grandchildren, or a perceived need to slow down in life may make caregiving seem like an impossible task. The timing is rarely ideal. The job description of a caregiver may read like this: must adapt to significant life changes and possess the ability to juggle balls and balance plates while assuring the health of another human being.

Don't go willy-nilly into caregiving without a strategy. Prepare yourself for this vitally important, yet underappreciated, work. Be ready for double-barreled challenges to your patience and temperament. Have a Teflon attitude toward comments made by those who have no way of knowing all that you do.

If, and when the 'switch' flips, realize this is not purposeful on the part of your loved one. Don't react, just go with the flow. Have your feet set firmly on the ground when feelings of burden and stress settle upon you. Remember the meaning of the word love. Find peace in the middle of turmoil, a place for meditation and prayer. Caregiving is immensely difficult. Your health and sense of well-being are essential for the cause.

There are rewards for the family caregiver. There will be darkness, but there will be warm, lasting light in the end. The loving care you have provided for your family member will define and reward you forever.

RESOURCES

Caregiving

Family Caregiver Alliance
National Center for Caregiving
785 Market Street, Suite 750
San Francisco, CA. 94103
(415) 434-3388
(800) 445-8106
http://www.caregiver.org/
info@caregiver.org

Center for Disease Control and Prevention;
Family Caregiving: The Facts
http://www.cdc.gov/aging/caregiving/facts.htm

AARP, 2008: Houser, A. et al, AARP Public Policy Institute,
Valuing the Invaluable: The Economic Value of Family Caregiving
http://www.aarp.org/politics-society/advocacy/caregiving-advocacy.html

NAC, 2006: National Alliance of Caregiving, Evercare Study of
Caregivers in Decline
http://www.caregiving.org/data/Caregivers

An excellent resource for links to many websites dealing with the
needs and issues of the family caregiver.
http://caring.com

The Spiritual Health of the Caregiver

The Caregiver's Voice
Spirituality Strengthening the Caregiver
Guest article by Dr. Carol Peters-Tanksley
03 March 2017
http://thecaregiversvoice.com

Dr. Carol Tanksley
http://www.drcarolministries.com

Respite Care

Respite Care-Eldercare Locator
http://www.eldercare.gov/Eldercare.NET/Public/Resources/Factsheets/Respite_Care.aspx

ARCH National Respite Network and Resource Center
http://archrespite.org

Where to Find Respite: Resources for Caregivers
https://AgingCare.com

Alzheimer's Disease

Alzheimer's Association
www.alz.org
This is an invaluable resource for anyone who cares for an individual with this disease. Information about support groups, caregiver, respite care, and the progression of the disease is given, along with the latest research concerning Alzheimer's disease.

Alzheimer's Disease: Unraveling the Mystery
Looking for the Causes of AD
Alzheimer's Disease Education and Resource Center

The Dying Process

Hospice Patient Alliance
http://www.hospicepatients.org

End of Life: Helping with Comfort and Care
National Institute of Health
National Institute on Aging
http://www.nia.nih.gov/

The Dying Process-Palliative Care
http://www.palliativecare.org/

When Someone You Love Stops Eating and Drinking
https://www.dignityhealth.org/content/cm/media/documents/stopse
atinganddrinking.pdf

Cerebral Vascular Accident

American Stroke Association
http://www.strokeassociation.org

American Heart Association
http://www.heart.org

REFERENCES

AM J Nurs, 2008 Sep; 108(9 suppl): 23-27

Bevans, Margaret, Sternberg, Esther. Caregiving Burden, Stress and Health Effects Among Family Caregivers of Adult Cancer Patients. JAMA, MA 2012 Jan 25, 307(4) 398-403

Brodaty, Henry, Donkin, Marika. Family caregivers of people with dementia. Dialogues Clin Neurosci, 2009 Jun: 11(2): 217-228

Haley, William. The Family Caregiver's Role in Alzheimer's Disease. Neurology, May 1997, vol 48 no 5 255-295

McCullagh, Emily, et al. Determinants of Caregiving Burden and Quality of life in Caregivers of Stroke Patients. Stroke, 2005;36:2181-2186

Olson, Nancy. Respite: A positive and Powerful Piece to Strengthening Families. Respite Care Association of Wisconsin

Peters-Tanksley, Dr. Carol. Spirituality Strengthening the Caregiver. The Caregiver's Voice. (website) March 2017

Schulz, Richard, Sherwood, Paula. Physical and Mental Effects of Family Caregiving.

Smith, Melinda, Kemp, Gina. Helpguide.org. Caregiving Stress and Burnout. May 2016. Acces July 1016.

Stirling, Christine, Dwan, C, Mckenzie, A. Why Carers Use Adult Day Respite: a mixed method case study. BMC Health Services Research. 2014 14:245

Wilborn-Lee, Betty. The Effects of Stress and Burden on Caregivers of Individuals with a Chronic Illness. Walden University ScholarWork.

ACKNOWLEDGEMENTS

First of all, I'd like to thank my parents for doing the best they knew how in raising my sister Patricia, my brother Thomas, and myself. We turned out pretty well thanks to them. Thanks to Patricia and Thomas and their spouses, James and Joyce, respectively, for their support during this project. Thank you to Joyce for designing such a beautiful cover.

Thank you, Judy Wallace, for your editing efforts in completing this book. It was no small task. Your assistance was invaluable. Also, thank you to Mary Andahl in this regard and passing this on to the "Magician" Brian for final formatting, design, and completion. Without your help, this would have very likely ended up in a drawer.

Thank you to the various individuals who read this work and validated its usefulness. This was of great encouragement to me. Thank you to my children, Breanna, Evan, and Kaitlyn for understanding, at a young age, the emotion of it all, and to their mother, Nikki for her love and assistance to Ma over the years.

I want to thank Paula, Ma's caregiver during the last two or so years of her life. You loved Ma and it showed in the work you did.

Lastly, thank you to Darlene Hopkins for the assistance, care, and affection you showed Ma. I will be forever thankful for what you did for her.

Cheers to Ma!

For comments or questions please feel free to contact me via email at **unforeseenjourney.com** and visit my website at **johnrochebooks.com**

www.ingramcontent.com/pod-product-compliance
Lightning Source LLC
Chambersburg PA
CBHW060041030426
42334CB00019B/2437